CRYSTAL GRIDS

HANDBOOK

USE THE POWER OF THE STONES FOR
HEALING AND MANIFESTATION

JUDY HALL

FAIR WINDS

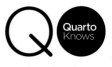

Inspiring | Educating | Creating | Entertaining

Brimming with creative inspiration, how-to projects, and useful information to enrich your everyday life, Quarto Knows is a favorite destination for those pursuing their interests and passions. Visit our site and dig deeper with our books into your area of interest: Quarto Creates, Quarto Cooks, Quarto Homes, Quarto Lives, Quarto Drives, Quarto Explores, Quarto Gifts, or Quarto Kids.

First Published in 2020 by The Harvard Common Press, an imprint of The Quarto Group,
100 Cummings Center, Suite 265-D, Beverly, MA 01915, USA.
T (978) 282-9590 F (978) 283-2742 QuartoKnows.com

The Harvard Common Press titles are also available at discount for retail, wholesale, promotional, and bulk purchase. For details, contact the Special Sales Manager by email at specialsales@quarto.com or by mail at The Quarto Group, Attn: Special Sales Manager, 100 Cummings Center, Suite 265-D, Beverly, MA 01915, USA.

24 23 22   4 5

ISBN: 978-1-59233-987-7

Digital edition published in 2020
eISBN: 978-1-63159-975-0

Library of Congress Cataloging-in-Publication Data available

Design: Samantha J. Bednarek
Page Layout: Samantha J. Bednarek
Illustration: Holly Neel
Photography: Michael Illas Photography, except pages 147 (bottom), 148 (bottom), 155 (bottom), 161 (bottom) by author; page 154 (both), 159 (bottom) by Jeni Campbell; pages 152 (top), 165 (top) , 159 (top), 163 (bottom), 164 (bottom), 149 (top), 157 (bottom), 167 (top), 146, 160 (bottom), 166 (top), 150 (bottom), 161 (top), 156 (top), 152 (bottom), 157 (top), 158 (bottom), 150 (top), 166 (bottom), 167 (bottom), 165 (bottom) by shutterstock.com

Printed in China

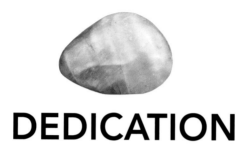

DEDICATION

To crystal lovers everywhere

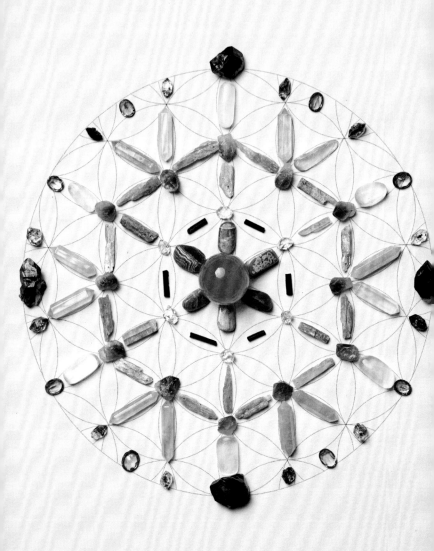

CONTENTS

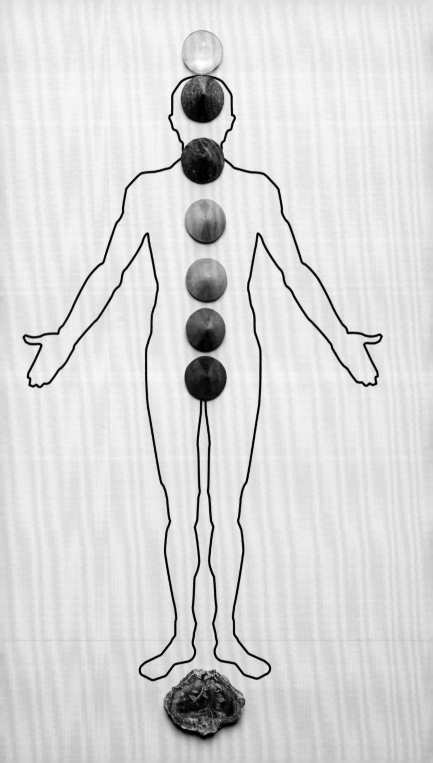

INTRODUCTION

CRYSTAL GRIDS synthesize powerful crystal vibrations and sacred geometric energy. To put it simply, they are energetic technology in action. Each grid has a unique harmonic resonance, and to stand inside a crystal grid is to experience the creative matrix of the universe made manifest. Being in the energy of a grid can be a vibrant event, profoundly energizing and expansive—or it can be a deeply peaceful experience that brings you to a point of stillness and ultimate union. It all depends on the intention of the individual grid.

Grids underpin our world. They are found throughout nature: in the perfect spiral of a sunflower or a pinecone; in the precise curves of an ammonite; in the cells of a honeycomb; or in the hidden beauty of a snowflake. They are the internal lattice structure of a crystal—and of the human body. Functioning rather like cosmic glue, grids support the visible and invisible worlds. In Drunvalo Melchizedek's words, they are the "architecture of the universe."

Crystal grids are potent tools because they harness nature's own manifestation energy. And combining several crystals into a grid has a far greater impact than placing one crystal alone. Whether a grid is created from a single type of crystal or from two or more types, the synergetic interaction of the crystal vibrations with the underlying forcefield, imbued with personal intent, becomes incredibly "power-full."

While a grid seems to be a flat, one-dimensional shape, it actually creates a multi-dimensional energetic net that expands throughout the space in which the grid is situated. This forcefield amps up your intention exponentially. A small triangular layout, for instance, energetically cleanses and protects a whole house, while a simple spiral radiates energy over a vast area or attracts abundant prosperity into its center. And a hexagram placed on a photograph energetically transfers healing to a person at a distance.

Placing your grid on a cloth or background of a complementary color enhances the power of your grid even further. Use natural base materials whenever possible, such as wood, linen, cotton, slate, or stone, as they will help anchor and actualize the grid's energies (although the color of a cloth is more important than the material from which it's made).

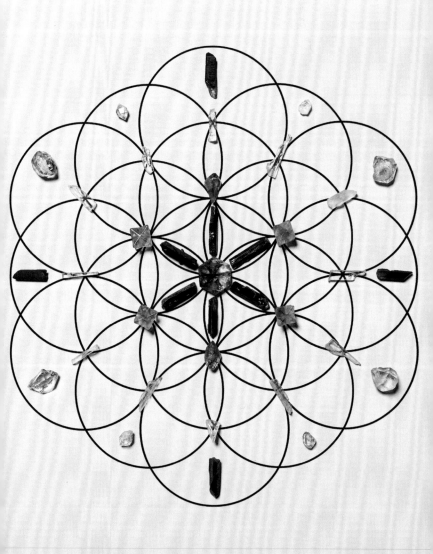

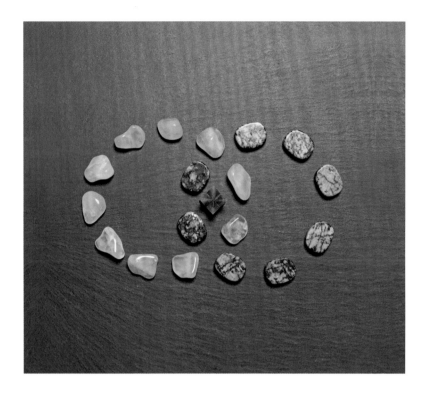

THE PURPOSE OF A GRID

The possibilities for a grid are endless. Grids can be large or small; they can be placed indoors, on or around your body, or in the environment. Remember that a grid's energetic net spreads way beyond the grid itself, so size is not an issue—a small one can be very powerful indeed. And grids offer countless benefits. They can create abundance, safeguard space, and neutralize toxic dross. They can attract love into your life or send forgiveness and healing intent. They can be set up for world peace, or to heal a devastated forest and the after-effects of a natural disaster.

Grids stabilize and cleanse energies, too. They're valued for their beneficial effects on the human energy field. Grids unblock and rebalance the aura, dispersing dis-ease (not to be confused with "disease") and creating well-being. They can be used for relaxation, emotional clearing, support, or deep healing, or for more specific outcomes, such as overcoming insomnia or headaches, or the detrimental effects of electromagnetic fields. Grids created for a specific outcome such as these can be left in place for long periods, provided that the crystals are regularly cleansed.

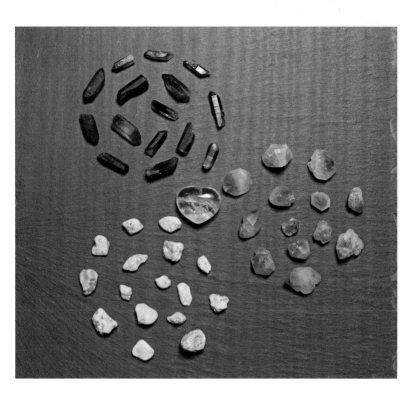

But there is no hard and fast rule for how long a grid needs to be left in place—or for which grid to choose. Trust yourself. Whichever grid shape appeals to you is the right grid for you. And whatever feels energetically *right* ensures the best outcome for you. Don't hesitate to experiment and modify the shape of a grid to suit your needs if your intuition tells you this would be more beneficial. When a grid has completed its work, thank it and then dismantle it.

Crystal Grid

Based on the subtle energy dynamics of sacred geometry, a crystal grid is a precise pattern laid using empowered crystals for the purpose of manifesting a desired outcome, or for cleansing and safeguarding a space.

INTENTION

Clear intention is the key to successful grid-working, as is maintaining that intent as the grid is set out. Intention is what empowers and activates the crystals and fires up the grid. Then, once it's activated, the grid is left to function without interference. But that doesn't mean that you can forget about your grid after you've laid and activated it. It's still important that you remain gently aware of how your intention is progressing over time—without constantly focusing on it or projecting it into the future—and that you cleanse your grid regularly. You'll know if you need to cleanse your grid—or rearrange the crystals or add or subtract appropriate ones—because you'll notice that energy begins to dissipate rather than build each day. If this occurs, cleanse your crystals, add or subtract appropriate crystals if necessary, and recharge them with intention. There is no set schedule for doing this. Simply remain aware of your intention and trust your intuition to tell you when your grid should be cleansed. (After cleansing, you may notice an immediate resurgence of the crystals' energy, or they may rebuild slowly as they shift to accommodate changes that have already occurred.)

INTUITION

Laying out grids helps you to develop your intuition: the "inner sight" that simply *knows*. Intuition helps you to recognize the appropriate placement for a crystal or exactly the right grid for your purpose, because intuition tunes into your body's innate, but largely unconscious until developed, ability to read energies. So, the more you rely on your intuition when selecting or using crystals, the stronger your intuition will become. In your crystal work, always go with your heart, the seat of the intuition, rather than your head.

USING THIS BOOK

This book is designed to be a roadmap, a guide to harnessing the phenomenal power of crystals, combined with sacred geometry. The more you use it, the more proficient you will become. So, every time you start a new project, lay a grid. Whenever you feel out of sorts, anxious, or ill at ease, lay a grid. If you have a desire to manifest an outcome, create a grid. If you want to protect your space, or to see peace in our world, build a grid. You'll find plenty of examples and grid-kit suggestions to guide you in this book. You can place your own crystals over those in the photographs or lay the grids on backgrounds that are appropriate for you. As you become more familiar with the technique, feel free to adapt the basic grids, or to use the more advanced grids, if you like. But whatever you do, activate your grids with focused intention—and then watch the results unfold with awe and gratitude.

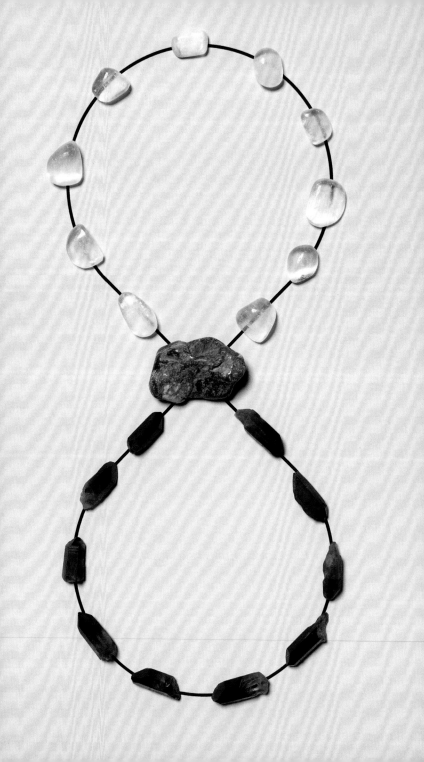

CHAPTER ONE

THE LANGUAGE OF CREATION

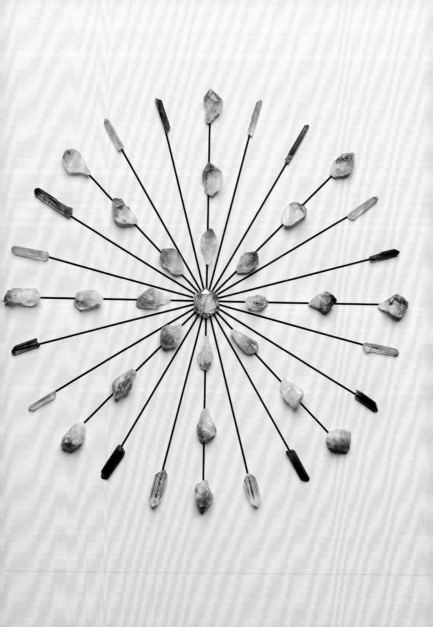

SACRED GEOMETRY

Sacred geometry is the archetypal structure of life—the form in which creation organizes itself, and the foundation on which the entire natural world is built. Through sacred geometry we discover the inherent proportion, balance, and harmony that exists in any situation, in all manifest reality, and in everyday life. Sacred geography, the interaction between sacred geometry and matter, describes the fundamental structure of space, time, and everything in between.

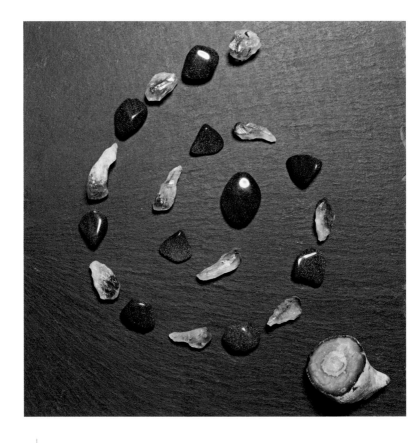

Basic Guide to Shapes

Virtually all sacred geometry is founded on simple, basic shapes that can be locked together in ever-increasing complexity. Each shape has a specific purpose and meaning:

- **Circle:** unity, completion, protection, boundary, initiation, healing

- **Triangle:** protection, manifestation, creation, integration

- **Square:** consolidation, stability, strength, protection

- **Spiral:** vortex energy, drawing in, radiating or releasing energy

- **Pyramid:** creation, rebirth, out-of-body journeying

- **Pentagon (five-sided polygon):** stability, clearing, completeness, the elements

- **Pentacle (five-pointed star):** drawing down energy, magical protection, connecting the elements

- **Hexagram (six-pointed star):** protection, energy balancing, consolidation, uniting heart and mind, above and below

- **Sphere:** encompassing all, inherently unstable

- **Cube:** limiting and delineating, inherently stable

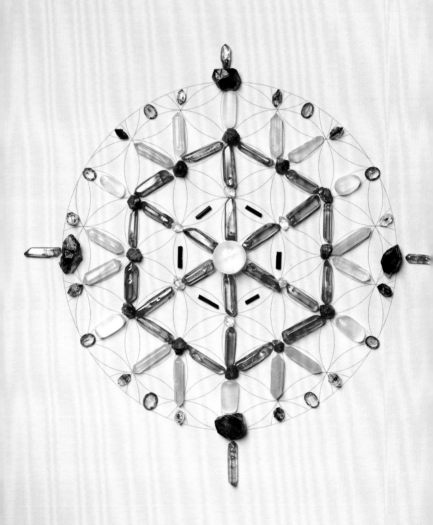

THE EFFECT OF COLOR

Color subtly alters the way a crystal functions in a grid. Vibrant "hot" colors energize and stimulate, while paler colors tend to be calming and "cool."

Transparent crystals may be either energizing or dissipating, as called for by the individual grid, harmonizing its energetics. Dark colors, on the other hand, transmute and ground energy. Black crystals, such as Smoky Quartz or Shungite, have a structure that captures energy as the light is absorbed. This means that the crystal draws in and holds toxic energies such as electromagnetic "smog," or ill-wishing. They also anchor the grid into the environment.

During crystal healing and grid work, some areas may need sedating and others may need stimulating. Choosing an appropriate color or colors of crystals harmonizes the energy flow.

CRYSTAL COLOR SPECTRUM

Black: Black crystals are strongly protective. They entrap negative energies that are then either neutralized or transmuted into positive energy. For this reason, they make excellent detoxifiers. They can also help to identify gifts that are hidden in the shadows—that is, they can help you to recognize potential and opportunities that you may not have been aware of before. Grids from black crystals ground the physical body and protect the environment.

Brown: Brown crystals resonate with the earth chakras. They are cleansing and purifying, grounding and protective. Use them to absorb toxic emanations and negative energies and to induce stability and centeredness. They are excellent for long-term use but need regular cleansing.

Silver-Gray: Metallic and silvery-gray crystals have alchemical properties of transmutation. That is, they convert negative energy into positive. They make excellent journeying crystals, traditionally imparting invisibility, helping the traveler to pass safely and unharmed. These crystals resonate with the earth chakras and are useful for shadow work. The shadow is a disowned, dejected, rejected, and isolated part of the overall self that tends to be denied, and so the shadow gets projected "out there" into external experiences. It forms an unconscious snag, thwarting our most well-meant intentions. Home to the wounds left over from childhood, ancestral trauma, and previous lives, the shadow also contains gifts that have been repressed. As crystals heal the energetic patterns that contain the wounds, it is not always necessary to connect to their source. Integrating the shadow through journeying, crystal work, or therapy opens up a new emotional vitality.

Gold: Gold stones have long been associated with abundance and manifestation, as they generate energy and also facilitate en*lighten*ment. Use them for long-term grids to draw prosperity and new vitality into your life.

Red: Red crystals resonate with the base and sacral chakras. They energize and activate, strengthening libido and stimulating creativity. Red crystals generate and circulate energy as required. This effect can be extremely stimulating, though, and may over-excite volatile emotions, so red crystals are best for short-term use.

Pink: Exceedingly gentle, pink crystals carry the essence of unconditional love and promote forgiveness. In grids, they attract more love into the seeker's life. They can provide comfort and alleviate anxiety, making them useful heart-healers. Pink crystals also help to overcome loss, release grief, and dispel trauma. Instilling acceptance, they resonate with the three-chambered heart chakra and are ideal for long-term use.

Peach: Gently energizing peach crystals unite the heart and sacral chakras, combining love with action. Use them in grids intended to help you move forward placidly in your life.

Orange: Orange crystals activate and release and are useful for building up energetic structures, since their energetic output locks together and does not dissipate. Many attract abundance. They stimulate creativity and increase assertiveness. An orange grid grounds projects into the physical world and gets things done. This color resonates with the sacral chakra.

Yellow: Yellow crystals work with the solar plexus, and the mind, balancing emotion and intellect; a yellow grid instills clarity. These grids are excellent for reducing seasonal depression, bringing the warmth of the sun into winter.

Green: Calming and cleansing, green crystals resonate with the heart chakra, providing emotional healing and instilling compassion and tranquility. They also draw higher consciousness down to earth, anchoring it. A green grid is useful when energy needs sedating or when emotions need pacifying.

Green-Blue and turquoise: These crystals resonate with higher levels of being, stimulating spiritual awareness and metaphysical abilities. Many turquoise crystals connect to cosmic consciousness, drawing it down to earth; all instill profound peace and relaxation. These crystals work at the third eye and soma chakras, uniting intuition and the heart.

Blue: Blue crystals resonate with the throat, third eye, soma, and causal vortex chakras, stimulating self-expression, facilitating communication, and linking to the highest states of consciousness. They ground or project spiritual energy and assist intuition and channeling. Traditionally, these crystals procured the assistance of spirits of light to counteract darkness. A blue grid stimulates intuition and metaphysical abilities, bringing about mystical perception.

Indigo: Indigo crystals link to the highest states of consciousness and to the most profound depths of space. With powerful spiritual awakening qualities, these crystals integrate and align, stimulating service to others. They can be useful for cooling over-heated energies, too. Stimulating intuition and metaphysical abilities, they bring about mystical perception of the world when placed at the third eye or soma chakras.

Lavender and purple: Purple crystals resonate with the higher crown chakras and multi-dimensional realities, drawing spiritual energy into the physical plane and encouraging service to others. Lavender and violet crystals have a lighter and finer vibration that links to the highest states of awareness.

Magenta: Magenta crystals link to the higher crown chakras, particularly the soul star and causal vortex, and stimulate connection to multi-dimensional realities. Use them to open the higher vibration chakras around the head to expand consciousness.

Clear or white: Clear crystals carry the vibration of pure light and higher consciousness. They resonate with the higher crown chakras. These crystals purify and focus energy, connecting the highest realms of being. Use them when situations need clarifying, or for opening intuition and gaining insight. Clear crystals are powerful energizers, radiating energy into the environment. In grids, they purify and heal the aura and physical body.

Combination and bi-colored crystals: Combination crystals create additional possibilities. Synergizing the qualities of component colors or crystals to work holistically together, they are often more effective than individual crystals, because their vibrations are raised to a higher energetic frequency.

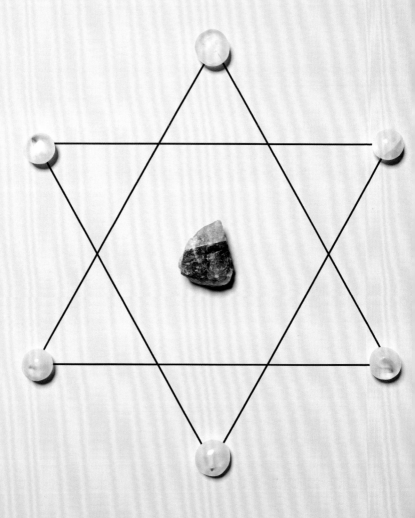

THE SCIENCE
OF SHAPE

Crystal shape takes two forms: internal and external. Both affect how energy moves through a grid. The internal geometric lattice of a crystal defines the system to which it belongs. This lattice, with its precise replication of internal facets and angles, remains the same, regardless of the crystal's external shape. It is found in even the tiniest piece, and it is replicated in the largest. So, a crystal can be tumbled, raw or faceted, flawless or chipped, small or large, and it still has the same effect—as indeed it does when it takes on apparently very different external forms.

A crystal's external shape, whether natural or achieved by cutting and polishing, doesn't affect its inherent properties; but, as we'll see, it does mediate how and where crystal energy flows.

UNIVERSAL BUILDING BLOCKS

At the heart of a crystal is its stable lattice. Within this structure, dynamic particles rotate in constant motion around a central point, generating energy. So, although a crystal may look outwardly serene, it is a seething molecular mass vibrating at a specific frequency—and generating energy. As the crystal frequency is stable and "pure," crystals entrain—that is, bring into balance—energy fields around them, which makes crystals extremely effective stabilizers. In this way, grids transform unstable energy patterns, such as those in the human body or its environment.

THE CRYSTAL SYSTEMS

Crystals are created from atoms that are packed together in an orderly fashion: the internal lattice. And individual crystals are recognizable by the way in which their component molecules fill the internal space. Each family of crystals has its own unique signature lattice. Under a microscope, a large, small, or differently colored example of the same crystal has the same makeup. It will, however, also belong to an overall crystal group, or "family." Each crystal system functions in a slightly different way, channeling energy according to the lattice. There are seven main crystal groups, plus the amorphous system. Solidified natural substances, such as Amber, are deemed amorphous.

The crystal systems are:

Amorphous or organic (no lattice): Amorphous energy surrounds and protects a body or a space. Energy flows rapidly and can be a catalyst for growth or can induce a cathartic release of toxicity.

Isometric (cubic): Stabilizes, grounds, and cleanses energy; releases tension and encourages creativity. Cubic crystals are excellent for grids that create structure and reorganization. This is the only crystal form that does not bend rays of light as they pass through it.

Hexagonal: Organizes and balances energy and provides support; useful for exploring specific issues.

Monoclinic: Increases perception and balances the systems of the body; useful for purification.

Orthorhombic: Vibrant and energetic; cleanses and dispels, increases the flow of information.

Tetragonal: Transformational; opens, harmonizes, and balances energy flow, and brings resolution.

Triclinic: Protective, integrating energy and opposites; opens perception, facilitating exploration of other dimensions.

Trigonal (hexagonal): Focuses and anchors energy, invigorates, and protects the aura and environment.

THE EFFECT OF EXTERNAL SHAPE

The outer form of a crystal, especially when it's artificially shaped, does not necessarily reflect its inner lattice, but it may subtly amend the way in which energy flows through it.

Ball: Emits energy equally all round. Forms a window to facilitate movement through time. Balls make an excellent centerpiece for a grid that radiates energy into the environment.

Cluster: Several points on a base radiate energy multi-directionally. These make a useful keystone for grids.

Double terminated: Points at both ends emit energy. Double terminations break old patterns and move energy in both directions through a grid.

Egg: Gently pointed end focuses energy. Rounded end radiates it more widely. Place point-down in a grid to channel energy into a body or the Earth, or place point-up to radiate it out.

Elestial: Folded with many terminations, windows, and inner planes, an elestial radiates gently flowing energy that opens the way to insight and change. These make a useful keystone or anchor for grids.

Faceted: Semi-precious and precious stones are often faceted to increase the amount of light penetrating the crystal, creating brilliance. This does not make them more effective for use in a grid: raw or tumbled stones work just as well.

Generator: Six-pointed end or several points radiating equally in all directions. Focuses healing energy or intention and draws people together.

Geode: Hollow cave-like formation amplifies, conserves, and slowly releases energy. Geodes are useful when energy is stagnant and needs constant, steady revitalization. They are also helpful where earth energy is flowing too fast and the grid has been placed to slow or redirect the flow.

Manifestation: A smaller crystal encased within an outer crystal. As its name suggests, it carries the power of manifestation, especially of abundance, but can be harnessed to any intention. Place a manifestation crystal as the keystone in an abundance grid.

Merkaba: A representation of divine "source" energy, a Merkaba is a star tetrahedron, a three-dimensional eight-pointed star created from two triangular pyramids, with one pointing up and the other down. It balances and harmonizes energy, stepping down cosmic vibrations and grounding them into the physical plane, uniting "above" with "below." It is the perfect shape for a keystone within a grid as it contains the potential for limitless creation and DNA healing.

Palmstone: Flat and rounded, a palmstone calms and soothes the mind. It serves as the perfect keystone of a grid to create what you most desire.

Phantom: Pointed inner pyramid breaks old patterns and raises vibrations. Place phantoms point-out in an environmental grid to break old patterns and point inward in a grid placed on a body for the same purpose.

Point: Naturally faced point draws off energy when pointed out from the body and draws energy in when pointed toward the body. Useful for cleansing and energizing a grid.

Pyramid: A pyramidal crystal creates energy and emits it from its point. Or, it can protect internal space. Pyramids make excellent keystones in grids.

Raw: A rough chunk of the natural crystal or stone. Works well in grids, since the artificial shaping of crystals can subtly amend the natural energetic flow of the crystal material. Raw chunks are also ideal for outdoor grids, as they do not scratch and can withstand the weather.

Scepter: These crystals formed around a central core rod are excellent tools for inputting power and restructuring. They activate a grid.

Square: Consolidating energy, a square grounds and anchors intention. Naturally occurring square crystals such as Pyrite draw off negative energy and transform it.

Tumbled: These gently rounded stones draw off negative energy or bring in positive energy. They are ideal for use in grids as they do not have to be direction specific.

Wand: The long-pointed or specially shaped crystals focus energy and draw it off or bring in energy, depending on which way the point is facing. Useful for joining crystals in a grid to activate the energetic net.

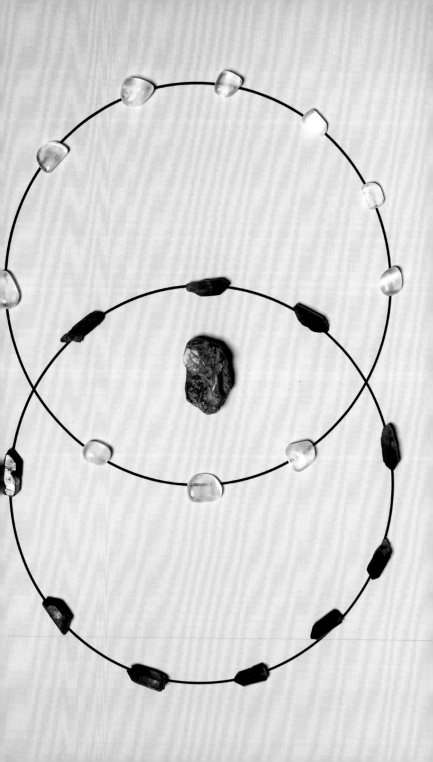

CHAPTER TWO

PREPARING AND SETTING UP A GRID

FINDING EXACTLY the right combination of crystals for your grid is the key to crystal power. While I offer suggestions in the grid-kits throughout this book, there's no need to feel limited by these suggestions. Use whichever crystals feel appropriate. You may well have crystals in your collection that would be perfect for your intention. This chapter will guide you to choose the right crystals to match your intention and will lay out the basic guidelines for setting up a grid. Finally, it will show you how to care for your crystals both before and after using them in a grid.

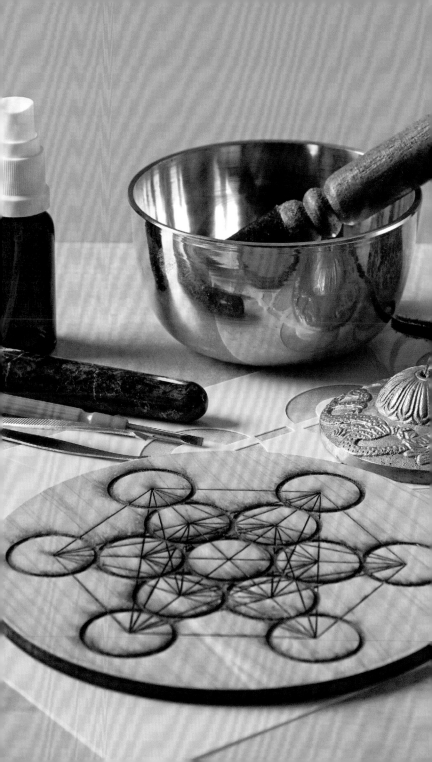

CRYSTAL SELECTION

It's not the outward beauty of a crystal that dictates its power; it's the crystal's individual properties.

You'll probably start by searching out crystals for the purpose for which you are setting up your grid. A photograph in this book may have caught your attention. If so, that's a good starting point. But where do you go from there—and what if you have no idea which crystals are appropriate for you right now? Put out the focused thought, "I'll find exactly the right crystals for me, now." Then run your fingers through a basket of crystals or pass your hand over the tubs that hold tumbled stones. There'll be several that "stick" to your fingers—or the shapes and energy of some crystals will just feel right. That's the intuitive approach. The kinesthetic intuitive approach is to dowse, as your body–mind already knows the answer.

If you prefer a reasoned, logical approach over an intuitive one, you could peruse the information on how colors, shapes, and specific grids mold the crystals' energy. Check out crystal reference books and seek crystals to match your intention.

When you've found a crystal, take a few moments to become attuned to it. Hold it in your hands, and feel its vibrations radiating into your core being. If those vibrations accord with your own, you'll feel calm and peaceful. If they are not, you'll begin to feel nauseous or jittery. If that's the case, you could choose another crystal, as the one you are holding may not be right for you at this time. This may also be an indication of inner work that you need to do, in which case scan through the personal grids.

If your crystal has a pointed end, face it in the direction in which the energy flows around the grid. Pointing a crystal inward draws in energy; pointing it out draws it off.

Wherever you find your crystals, make sure you cleanse and empower them before use.

Empathy Nicks and Self-Healed Crystals

Crystals for use in grids do not have to be perfect. In fact, points that are chipped or crystals that appear misshapen may work extra hard, as they empathize with wounds and pain and will apply their compassionate healing properties in the grid. "Self-healed" crystals exhibit internal breaks that have healed over time as the crystal continued to grow. Such crystals are particularly useful in healing grids.

CRYSTAL CARE

Crystals constantly pick up energy in addition to radiating it out. This is especially so when grids are left in place for a long period of time. That means your crystals need regular cleansing. Always start your grid with "clean" crystals. Keep the grid cleansed and recharged during its operation. Otherwise, the grid begins to emit detrimental, rather than beneficial, energy as it slowly runs out of steam, especially when it has been transmuting negative energies.

How often you cleanse your crystals depends on the purpose of the grid and on the intensity of the energy being absorbed or radiated. For example, protective and clearing grids need cleansing more frequently than those that attract abundance, love, and so on. Ultimately, there is no set rule as to timing, except to cleanse frequently, and to cleanse and recharge whenever the crystals begin to look "dull" and the grid is no longer working. Simply placing your hand over the grid will tell you whether the energy is bright and active or sluggish and in need of a reboot. Crystals also require purifying when the grid is dismantled.

INITIAL CRYSTAL CLEANSING

"The sound created by a singing bowl, tingshaws, a gong, or tuning fork is a pure vibration that cleanses and restores all crystals. If using a bowl, several crystals can be put in at once, enough to cover the bottom but not restrict the vibration. Tingshaws and a gong can be struck over several whilst a tuning fork can be struck and applied individually. Whatever you are using, listen carefully, and you will hear when the cleaning and charging is complete, as the sound will be clear and bright." —Terrie Celest, www.astrologywise.co.uk

TIP:
To smudge a crystal, hold it in the smoke from an incense stick or smudge bundle for a few moments, ensuring that all sides receive the smoke.

If the crystals are robust—that is, unless they are layered, fragile, soluble, or have tiny crystals on a matrix—cleanse them in running water, then place them in the sun or moonlight to recharge. If they are less robust, place them in brown rice overnight, smudge them with sweetgrass or incense, or use a singing bowl or tingshaws. Then place them in the sun or on a crystal to recharge. If the grid is to be buried in the ground, soak the keystone in Petaltone Z14 essence before covering, as the clearing effect lasts for several months. Otherwise, leave one crystal above the ground so that it can be sprayed regularly.

Once your grid is in place, lightly spray it with crystal clearing and recharge essence weekly or whenever the energy feels depleted or stagnant.

RECHARGING YOUR CRYSTALS

Place a crystal in the sun or moonlight for a few hours to recharge it or spray it with recharging essence. Placing crystals on large energizing crystals such as Carnelian or Quartz will also recharge your grids. (You may need to remove the crystals for a short time in order to do this.) If the grid is to be buried, leave one of the stones poking above ground to receive the sun's rays. Or spray with a recharging essence once cleansed.

GRID CLEARING AND RECHARGE ESSENCE

Ready-made crystal clearing essence sprays cleanse crystals and are especially useful for a grid that remains in place, as you don't need to move the crystals to cleanse them. You can also make your own cleansing and recharge spray. This essence also closes down the space after a grid has been deactivated and the crystals removed, which is not usually a function of ready-made sprays.

CRYSTAL CLEANSING AND RECHARGE SPRAY

To make your own crystal cleansing and recharge spray, you will need:

CLEARING

- Black Tourmaline
- Blue or Black Kyanite
- Hematite
- Shungite
- Smoky Quartz

RECHARGING

- Anandalite™
- Carnelian
- Golden Healer Quartz
- Citrine
- Orange Kyanite
- Quartz
- Red Jasper
- Selenite (use tumbled)

TOOLS

- Small glass bowl
- Spring water
- Small glass bottle
- Funnel
- Spray bottle
- Frankincense, lavender, sage, or a similar essential oil
- Vodka or white rum

DIRECTIONS

1. Select one or two crystals from the clearing list and one or two from the recharging list on the left. Ensure that the crystals are thoroughly cleansed.
2. Hold them in your hands for a few moments and ask them to cleanse the grid, your crystals, or your space.
3. Place the crystals in a small glass bowl and cover with spring water. (Use fresh water from a pure source; avoid tap water or only use it when nothing else is available. If you do use tap water, include raw Shungite in the crystal mix.)
4. Place the bowl in sunlight for a few hours. Cover if necessary.
5. Remove the crystals and, using a funnel, pour the water into a glass bottle. Fill it one-third full.
6. Add a few drops of essential oil, such as frankincense, sage, or lavender, and top up the bottle with vodka or white rum, which will act as a preservative. This is the mother essence.
7. Label the bottle with the date and contents. You can use it immediately or store it in a cool place for several months.
8. Fill the spray bottle with spring water. Add seven drops of the mother essence. Label it.
9. Spray the grid from above, lightly misting all the crystals.

SETTING UP YOUR GRID

BASIC GRID-KIT

If you have a few basic cleansed gridding crystals on hand, you can set up a grid instantly. Choose six equal-sized crystals, or as many as the grid requires, and a larger one for the keystone. A varied selection of crystals is best, but don't overdo the number—three or four types are probably enough. Choose the ones that resonate with you from the following list.

Grounding and anchoring: Boji Stones, Flint, Granite, Hematite, Obsidian, Petrified Wood, Smoky Quartz, Brown Carnelian, Polychrome Jasper, Mookaite Jasper, Picture Jasper

Protective: Amber, Amethyst, Apache Tear, Black Tourmaline, Green Aventurine, Herkimer Diamond, Labradorite, Lepidolite, Shungite, Smoky Quartz, Mookaite Jasper, Porcelain Jasper

Cleansing: Amethyst, Apache Tear, Calcite, Chlorite Quartz, Flint, Halite, Obsidian, Quartz, Selenite, Shungite, Smoky Quartz

Energizing: Carnelian, Citrine, Herkimer Diamond, Lemurian Seed, Quartz, Red Jasper, Imperial Topaz, Sunstone, Ruby, Garnet

Abundance: Carnelian, Citrine, Goldstone, Jade, Tiger's Eye, Topaz

Personal healing: Bloodstone, Quantum Quattro Silica, Que Sera (Llanoite/Vulcanite), Emerald, Shungite, Golden Healer

Environmental healing: Aragonite, Kambaba Jasper, Petrified Wood, Rhodozite, Rose Quartz, Shungite, Smoky Quartz

High-vibration, light-bringing: Anandalite™ (Aurora Quartz), Celtic Quartz, Lemurian Seed, Moldavite, Petalite, Phenacite, Selenite, Trigonic Quartz

Intuitive: Apophyllite, Azurite, Bytownite, Herkimer Diamond, Blue or Green Kyanite, Labradorite, Lapis Lazuli, Larimar, Clear Quartz, Rhomboid Selenite, Selenite, Tangerine Aura Quartz

DOES SIZE MATTER?

It most emphatically does not. Again, when it comes to crystals, the biggest and most beautiful does not equal the most powerful. And while it makes sense to place large crystals where they can be seen if they are to be left in situ, so that they remain undisturbed, smaller or rough pieces work equally well in grids. That's because all crystals of a specific type are connected by what Michael Eastwood, an English crystal authority, calls "the crystal oversouls," which is a unified field of consciousness that interconnects the individual crystals of that type, wherever they may be. The smaller ones take their power from the whole. If you wish, you can place smaller crystals on a larger one of the same type before use to boost their connection to the oversoul power, but this is by no means essential.

DOWSING FOR YOUR CRYSTALS

Dowsing is an easily learned skill that assists not only in selecting crystals, but also in choosing the appropriate grid for your purpose, and in figuring out where to position it. You can use a pendulum or finger dowse, whichever you prefer. Neither method is "better" than the other. It is a matter of personal preference and finding which works for you. Each method accesses the ability of your intuitive body–mind connection to tune into subtle vibrations and to influence your hands. A focused mind, trust in the process, and clear intent supports your dowsing.

PENDULUM DOWSING

If you are familiar with pendulum dowsing, use the pendulum in your usual way. If you are not familiar with it, pendulum dowsing is an easy skill to learn. It will assist in placing crystals within a grid, positioning the grid itself, and in establishing how long to leave a grid in place or whether it needs amending from time to time. Pendulum dowsing is particularly useful when placing large outdoor grids or crystals on maps. To pendulum dowse:

1. Hold your pendulum between the thumb and forefinger of your most receptive hand with about a hand's length of chain hanging down to the pendulum. You'll soon recognize a length that's comfortable for you.

2. Wrap the remaining chain around your fingers so that it does not obstruct the dowsing. Tuck your arm into your side, bend your elbow, and hold out your hand at a right angle to your upper arm.

3. Ascertain your "yes" and "no" responses. Some people find that the pendulum swings in one direction for "yes" and at right angles to that axis for "no," while others have a backward and forward swing for one reply, and a circular motion for the other.

4. A "wobble" of the pendulum indicates "maybe," or that it is not appropriate to dowse at that time. Ask whether dowsing is appropriate, and if the answer is "yes," check that you are asking the right question. If the pendulum stops completely, this indicates that it is inappropriate to ask at that time.

5. Understand your particular pendulum response by holding the pendulum over your knee and asking, "Is my name [give your name]?" The direction that the pendulum swings indicates "yes." Check by asking, "Is my name [give incorrect name]?" to establish "no." Or, program in "yes" and "no" by swinging the pendulum in a particular direction a few times, saying as you do so: "This is 'yes'," and swinging it in a different direction to program "no."

Hold the pendulum in your most receptive hand. Slowly run your finger along the list of possible crystals in the grid-kit suggestions, noting whether you get a "yes" or "no" response. You could also dowse over the illustrations throughout this book, in other crystal books, or in a crystal shop. Check the whole kit to see which "yes" response is strongest, as there may well be several that could be appropriate, or you may need to use several crystals in combination. Another way to do this, if you have a selection of crystals available, is to touch each crystal in turn, again noting the "yes" or "no" response that results.

Your pendulum can pinpoint the exact placement for a crystal, which is especially useful when creating large outdoor grids. However, there may be times when a crystal displays a mind of its own and constantly shifts its position slightly out of alignment within the grid. If this is the case, allow the crystal to settle itself, which will open up a space for new possibilities to unfold.

A pendulum can also be used to establish how long you should leave a grid in place. Some grids may only need to be left in place for a minute or two before being dismantled or rearranged with fresh crystals. First, ask whether the period required is minutes, hours, days, weeks, or months. When you have gotten the answer, ask, "One minute [or hour, day, week, or month]? Two minutes [or hours, days, weeks, or months]?" and so on, until the length of time has been ascertained.

FINGER DOWSING

Finger dowsing answers "yes" and "no" questions quickly and unambiguously, and it can be done unobtrusively in situations in which a using pendulum might provoke unwanted attention. This method of dowsing works particularly well for people who are kinesthetic—that is, whose bodies respond intuitively to subtle feelings—but anyone can learn to finger dowse. To finger dowse:

1. Hold the thumb and first finger of your right hand together.
2. Then loop the thumb and finger of your left hand through the first "loop" to make a "chain."
3. Ask clearly and unambiguously whether this is the best and most appropriate crystal for your purpose. Either speak it aloud or within your mind.
4. Now pull gently but firmly. If the chain breaks, the answer is "no." If it holds, the answer is "yes."

Asking about periods of time requires a slightly different method for finger dowsing. First, ask whether the period required is minutes, hours, days, weeks, or months. When you have gained the answer, slot your fingers together and ask that they hold until the right answer is reached, then release. Then ask, "One minute [or hour, day, week, or month]? Two minutes [or hours, days, weeks, or months]?" and so on, until the length of time has been ascertained.

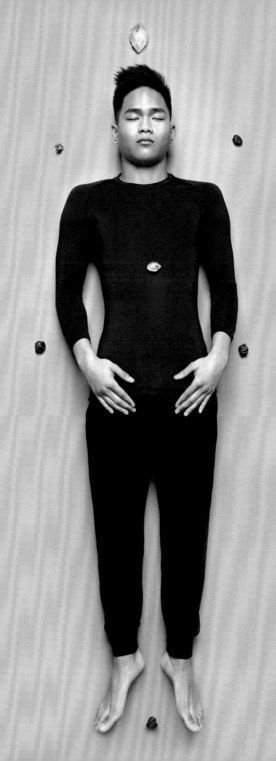

EMPOWERING YOUR CRYSTALS WITH INTENTION

To activate your crystals and imbue them with intention, simply hold the cleansed crystals in your hands, focus your attention on them, and say aloud:

I dedicate these crystals to the highest good of all and ask that their power be activated now to work in harmony with my focused intention. I also ask that the grid when assembled will [add your specific purpose for the grid], together with anything else that is appropriate at the highest level.

Remember to restate your intention when you lay the grid.

CHOOSING A LOCATION

The location for your grid needs to be appropriate for your intention and for the period it is to remain in place. Grids on or around your body are limited, although a grid can be placed around or under a bed, and the energetic effect will continue as a result. Small grids can be left in place in the home or workplace. Bigger grids can be left in place if they will not be disturbed and are accessible for cleansing. Choose a position appropriate to the space that will not be disturbed.

Grids can be placed in the following locations:

On or around your body
In your home or workspace
In the environment
Buried in the ground
On a photograph
On a map

HEALING CHALLENGE

When you're working with grids, a healing challenge—a period during which symptoms or situations initially worsen—may occasionally occur. If this happens while you're laying out or lying within a grid, remove yourself and hold detoxifying and restabilizing crystals such as Black Tourmaline, Shungite, Smoky Quartz, Flint, or Hematite. Place one at your feet until the situation settles. Before re-entering or returning to laying the grid, check by dowsing or by using intuition to see whether any crystals need to be removed or replaced. When you re-enter the grid, place a grounding and detoxifying crystal at your feet. If the grid has been laid in the environment—including a small grid laid in a room in your house—create a circle around it with the same crystals, or temporarily replace the keystone or anchor crystals with a detoxifying crystal. When the situation has settled, check that the correct crystals are in place. Replace any that have completed their work.

CHOOSING A GRID TEMPLATE

Match the shape of the grid to your intention and to the space available. If you are a beginner, start with one of the basic shapes, or try an example grid for a specific purpose. As you become familiar with grid energy, choose one of the more complex shapes, or create your own. Don't hesitate to amend or expand a grid that appeals to you. As you will see, some of the specific grids later in this book use variations of a basic template. But, remember that grids do not have to be complicated to be effective.

ALIGNING A GRID

Aligning your grid with the magnetic points of the compass draws in the power of the directions to assist in the work. Aligning a grid north to south smooths the energy flow, for instance, but you can also align it to sun- or moonrise, which varies throughout the year. Sun-orientated grids are active and initiating, while moon-orientated grids are nurturing and initiatory. It is also possible to align your grids in accordance with the traditional associations of the shamanic directions as follows:

North: Knowledge, restructuring, calming discord
South: Cleansing, flowing, and activating
East: Conception, removes strife, motivates new projects
West: Letting go, clearing, growth, renewal, rebirth
Above: Cosmic energy and light, energizing, the divine masculine
Below: Earthing, grounding, nurturing, the divine feminine

THE KEYSTONE

A point of power, a keystone focuses and amplifies the grid. It is usually the central stone, symbolizing the source of life. The keystone channels universal life force (Qi) to the grid, and its energy is then amplified by the grid. Quartz in its various forms is an ideal keystone, as it constantly transmutes, generates, amplifies, and radiates energy.

THE ANCHORS

Anchor stones hold the energy of a grid in place, grounding and centering it. They may be situated at or outside the corners of a square grid, for instance, or within the grid structure itself. Stones such as Flint, Aragonite, Smoky Quartz, or Granite make excellent anchor stones. Flint, Black Tourmaline and Shungite anchor a cleansing or high-vibration crystal grid, channeling transmuted energy down through the multi-dimensions to the Earth itself.

THE PERIMETER

A perimeter keeps the energies of a grid free from interference or disruption. It is not necessarily an integral part of the grid itself—although in some cases, it may be. (Perimeters may be important for a grid that's intended to contain energy and create a boundary, such as protecting a space; clearing electromagnetic fields [EMFs] in a house; creating a safe space; or inviting in a higher presence.) Quartz, in one of its many forms, is an ideal perimeter, as is Black Tourmaline or Shungite; they ground the grid into everyday reality. Triclinic crystals, such as Kyanite or Labradorite, or orthorhombic crystals such as Aragonite, make useful boundary stones, while Selenite creates a protective perimeter of light.

LAYING A GRID

1. Select your location.
2. Choose a place and time where and when you will not be disturbed.
3. Cleanse the space on which your grid will be laid.
4. Choose an appropriate background and color on which to lay your grid.
5. Gather your crystals together and thoroughly cleanse them.
6. Hold them in your hands and state your intention for the grid. Be specific and precise. You might say, "Please protect me and my space," for example.
7. Mark your template or use the examples in this book as a guide. Remember to orientate the grid appropriately. If your grid is intended to draw energy in or to provide protection, place the outermost crystals first. If your grid is intended to radiate energy, place the keystone first.
8. Check that the crystals are properly aligned. But note that if a crystal continually shifts its position, this may be to open up the unrecognized potential of a grid rather than restricting it to your immediate intention. If this occurs, leave the crystal where it wishes to settle.
9. Join up all the points to activate the grid with the power of your mind or a crystal wand.
10. Add a perimeter or anchor stones if appropriate.

TIP:
Handle small crystals with tweezers to make the placement more exact.

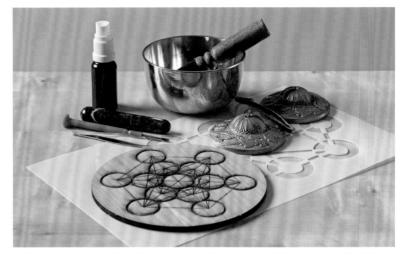

1. Gather the tools you will need for laying out and cleansing your grid. Tweezers and a flat blade such as a screwdriver assist in aligning the crystals.

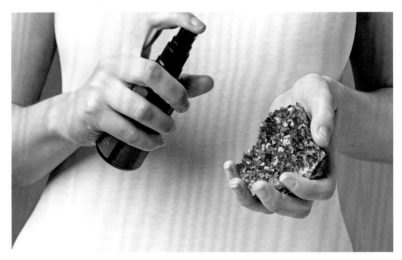

2. Cleanse your crystal thoroughly before use.

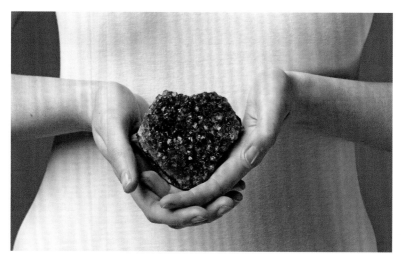

3. State your intention for the grid while holding the crystal.

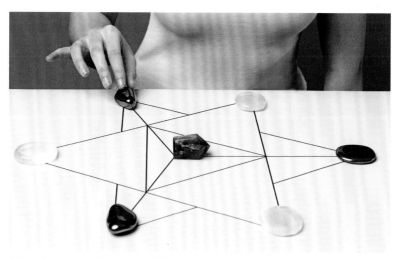

4. Place the major crystals within the grid.

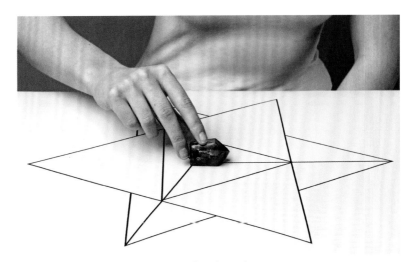

5. Place the keystone in the center of the grid first when radiating energy out.

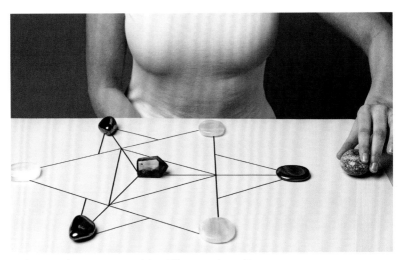

6. Place an anchor stone to ground the grid into everyday reality.

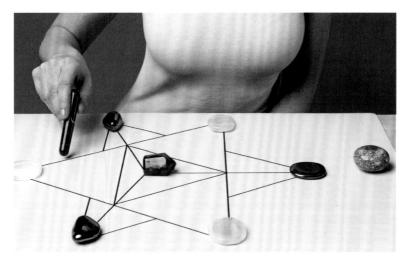

7. Join up the grid with a crystal wand or the power of your mind.

ACTIVATING THE GRID

To activate a grid once it has been laid, use a crystal wand or the power of your mind to join up all the points, including the keystone. If the grid does not have connecting lines to each crystal, take the wand (or your mind) into the central point and out again, touching each crystal in turn and weaving the energy into being. Finally, place the wand on the keystone and restate your intention.

KEEPING THE GRID ACTIVE

Check in with your grid on a regular basis (but don't overdo it!). How often you should check in with your grid depends on its purpose. Some, such as protective or transmuting grids, need daily checking, while outdoor grids or those set to attract abundance can happily be left alone for a week. To keep your grid active, restate your intention, cleanse the crystals if necessary, and remove or add further crystals if appropriate. But don't interfere with your grid too frequently, or you won't really give it a chance to work.

DISMANTLING THE GRID

Once a grid has served its purpose, it can be dismantled. Leaving activated crystals or the imprint of a grid lying around—especially if you go on to create other grids—can create an energetic cacophony. To deactivate a grid, cleanse the crystals thoroughly after dismantling (dark and smoky transmuting crystals may benefit from being buried in the Earth for a short time if they have been working particularly hard, or from being placed in uncooked brown rice overnight). Then hold the crystals in your hands, saying:

I thank these crystals for their work, which is no longer needed at this time. I ask that the power be closed until reactivated.

Put the crystals in sunlight and/or moonlight to recharge for a few hours or overnight, then place them in a box or a drawer. This effectively puts the crystals to "sleep" until they are required again.

Spray the space in which the grid was laid out with clearing and recharging essence. Some layouts create an extremely powerful multi-level energetic imprint that remains long after the grid has been dismantled. While grid imprints with a generalized purpose, such as bringing peace and tranquility or to render support, can be left to dissipate on their own, if a grid has been constructed to alleviate a specific situation or transmute a condition that has now passed, it may need specific energetic deconstruction. This deconstruction is especially necessary if you are using high-vibration crystals.

Sound is excellent for closing down such energetic imprints. You may need to sound a drum, singing bowl, tuning forks, or tingshaws over the space to completely close down the grid at all levels. Alternatively, you can smudge the space with sage or sweetgrass.

CUSTOM GRIDS

Once you understand the basic processes and energetic harmonics of grids, you can move on to creating your own. These grids don't need to be complex. A simple heart-shaped grid, for instance, is a potent way to draw love into your life—or to send it into the world. Custom grids can also be created to send healing to a person or to a place. Or, you may see a shape that appeals to you and inspires you to create a grid. Simply picture the grid with your mind, or dowse for the position of the crystals, following the procedures for laying a grid.

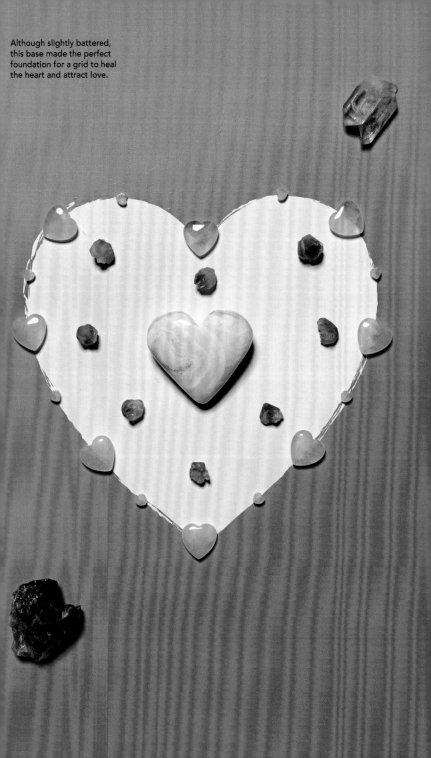

Although slightly battered, this base made the perfect foundation for a grid to heal the heart and attract love.

CHAPTER THREE

BASIC GRIDS

THE GRIDS IN THIS SECTION are simple, often requiring only a handful of crystals. Nevertheless, they are extremely powerful. And, as you'll see, some basic grids can be extended into other more complex, equally potent forms.

In most cases, there will be no set number of crystals or way to lay a grid. The number of crystals in a grid will vary according to their size and properties, and with the way in which they align with your intention—and with each other. Use your intuition or dowse to find the type and number of crystals to assist you in a particular grid—and to determine which grid is right for your purpose. Sometimes the crystals will deliberately move out of alignment to create a space for something new to emerge. The grids may need to have slight imperfections in the energetic net to allow change to take place and

possibilities to open up. If the grids are always precise and static, the outcome will always be the same. But opening a slightly "flawed" space activates the potential for what I always ask of a grid—"that or something better"—which I add to my intention statement. Crystals are wise, intelligent beings; they can see a lot further than we humans can. I've learned that if a crystal constantly shifts its position in the grid, it's saying, "This is where I need to be." If it falls on the floor, it may be saying, "Choose another crystal." Listen to the crystals rather than following the rules. The more you work with crystals and grids, the more your skills will develop, so you'll soon be able to sense crystals' energetic effects and intuitively know what a grid requires. Finally, remember to always use cleansed and dedicated crystals for your grids.

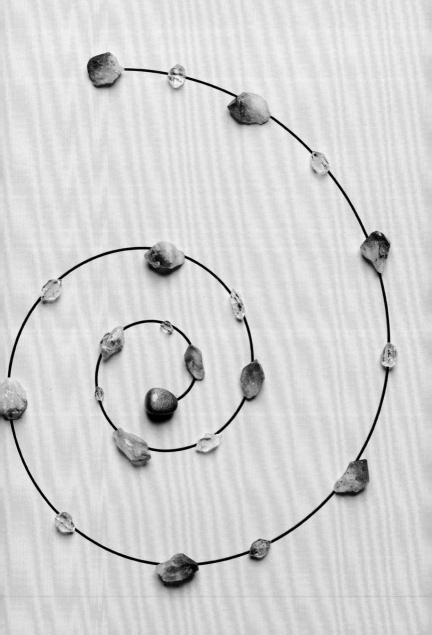

VESICA PISCIS

CREATION AND MANIFESTATION

A mystical conjunction, the Vesica Piscis is consciousness knowing itself and taking on form. This grid represents both unity and common ground, but the shape also represents separation into component parts. It is the start of life, thus the sphere of creation and manifestation.

Form: The Vesica Piscis is formed from two intersecting circles aligned so that the circumference of one circle touches the center point of the other. The circle is the simplest and most profound of forms, for it has no beginning and no end, and encompasses all possibilities. It is the ultimate expression of unity. Overlap the circles, however, and the Vesica Piscis gives birth to the triangle, the square, the hexagon, the Seed of Life, and the Flower of Life.

Uses: Lay the grid upright to draw energy down, or lay it sideways to integrate or to create energy. A symbol of unification and harmony, the Vesica Piscis bridges the spiritual and the physical. It blends logic, intuition, and emotion, or past, present, and future. This grid is excellent for conception, collaboration, conflict resolution, and finding common ground. It is extremely helpful when starting new ventures. Place a keystone in the center to symbolize your purpose.

Timing: Spring is ideal. Place the Vesica Piscis at a new moon when you're starting a fresh venture. A full moon is the most providential for conflict resolution and the integration of opposing forces, but this grid can be placed immediately if you encounter a crisis.

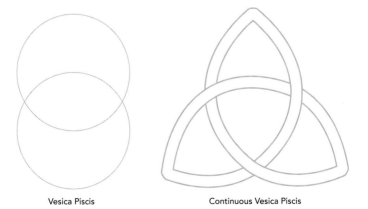

Vesica Piscis   Continuous Vesica Piscis

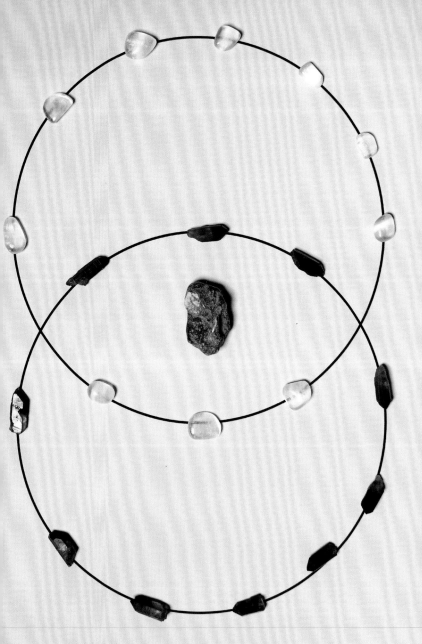

A simple circle of Smoky Quartz cleanses the energy and another
of Selenite infuses light, creating a Vesica Piscis. The keystone, Eye of the Storm
(Judy's Jasper), keeps the space calm and clear.

YOU WILL NEED:

- Sufficient crystals to create both circles
- Keystone

TO LAY THE GRID:

1. Hold your crystals in your hands and state your intention for the grid.
2. Lay the left-hand or bottom circle first, carefully aligning the crystals around the circle.
3. Lay the right-hand or top circle.
4. Place your keystone in the center, stating your intention once more.
5. Join the circles with a wand or the power of your mind.
6. When you're ready, dismantle the grid.

CONTINUOUS VESICA PISCIS

Place your crystals from the top point down and place a keystone in the central portion of the grid. Anchor stones at the bottom corners ground the energy into place.

Grid-kit suggestions: Grounding and anchoring crystals for the left-hand or bottom circle; high-vibration light-bringing crystals for the right-hand or top circle. Eye of the Storm (Judy's Jasper), Rose Quartz, Smoky Quartz, or Menalite for fertility

LEMNISCATE

GROUNDING AND UNIFYING

The lemniscate is a symbol of infinity, wholeness, and completion. The loops also reflect the balance of opposites: male and female, day and night, dark and light. This symbol also depicts perpetual motion and the interaction of energy and matter—that is, their indestructibility and their potential for transmutation. The term "infinity" was derived from the Latin word *infinitas*, which translates as "unboundedness." Indeed, this grid can be energetically expanded without limit.

Form: The lemniscate is composed of two circles in the same plane, drawn with a continuous line to create a figure of eight. It is a "seesaw" of clockwise and counterclockwise loops with a balance point in the center. The lemniscate can be used pointing upward to draw energy to a central point or placed sideways to create a continuous flow.

Uses: The lemniscate is an excellent rebalancing layout, particularly suited for placement on and around the human body. The grid both cleanses and draws in light to fill the vacuum created by the release of toxic energies. It can be used for situations in which two separate parts need to be drawn together, since infinity includes all time—past, present, and future—centered in the "now." The lemniscate grid actualizes intention into the present moment. Lay clearing crystals on the lower half and light-bringers on the top loop, and use over the heart seed, heart, and higher heart chakras as an immune stimulator or soother.

Timing: No special timing.

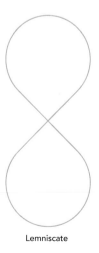

Lemniscate

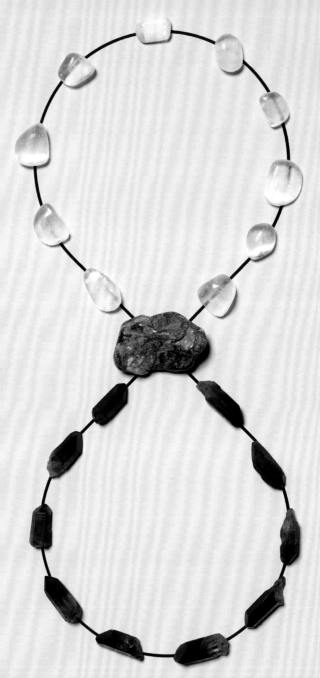

Selenite above Smoky Quartz linked by an Eye of the Storm (Judy's Jasper) keystone that also acts as a stabilizing anchor.

YOU WILL NEED:

- Sufficient cleansing and light-bringing crystals for each loop
- An appropriate keystone for the crossing point
- If using around or on the body, a grounding anchor stone

TO LAY THE GRID:

1. Hold your crystals in your hands and state your intention for the grid.
2. If you're laying the grid around your own body, ask an assistant to place the crystals for you.
3. Either place the keystone on your navel or in the center of the grid.
4. Lay the lower loop with cleansing and grounding crystals.
5. Lay the upper loop with energizing and light-bringing crystals.
6. Join up the grid with a crystal wand or the power of your mind.
7. When you're ready, dismantle the grid.

Grid-kit suggestions: Grounding and anchoring crystals for the left-hand or upper circle; high-vibration light-bringing crystals for the right-hand or lower circle. Mookaite Jasper, Porcelain Jasper

Heart grid: Emerald or Fuchsite for the upper circle; Lepidolite or Ruby for the base

TRIANGLE

TRANQUILITY, PROTECTION, AND MANIFESTATION

A triangle represents that which is solid, substantial, and complete in itself. As a grid, however, it not only protects that which is inside it—making it a useful protection mechanism—but also radiates energy out to fill a space and transmute energies. Triangular grids are excellent for smoothing discord and instilling the strength to overcome. A triangular grid can replicate itself endlessly.

Form: Triangles have three sides and three angles but take several forms. An equilateral triangle has equal sides and angles; an isosceles triangle has two equal sides and two equal angles; and a scalene triangle has three unequal sides and three unequal angles. The Golden Triangle is generated from the Golden Ratio spiral. The angles and sides arising from the shortest side are equal.

Uses: Excellent for protecting a space, triangular grids can be laid wherever there is disharmony, where protection is required, or where energy requires transmutation. It expands to fill the space, so it is particularly effective for small, long-term grids. A triangular grid blends logic, intuition, and emotion; mind, body, and spirit; past, present, and future; thought, word, and deed.

Timing: Lay your triangular grid as required. Replenish and cleanse at new and full moon.

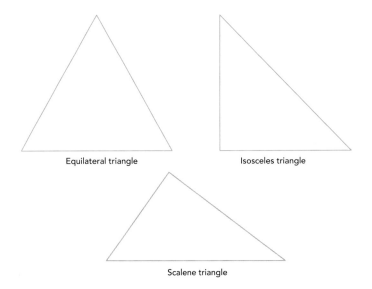

Equilateral triangle

Isosceles triangle

Scalene triangle

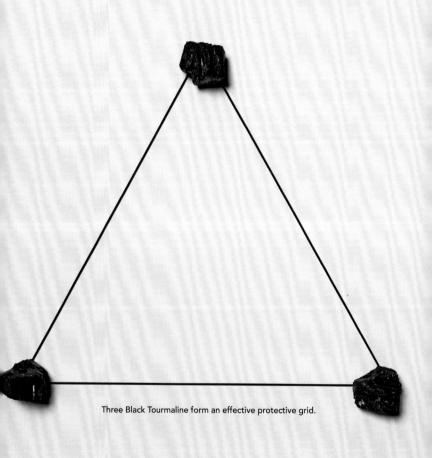

Three Black Tourmaline form an effective protective grid.

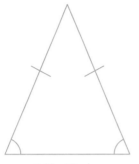

Golden Triangle

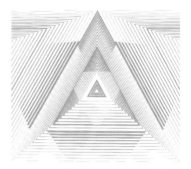

Energetic effect. In a triangular grid, the energy builds and expands both inward and outward to fill the whole space and create a protective energy field around the area.

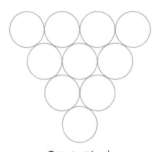

Tetractys triangle

YOU WILL NEED:

- Three fairly large, appropriate grid crystals

TO LAY THE GRID:

1. Hold your crystals in your hands and state your intention for the grid.
2. If protecting your space, place one crystal centrally along a wall or boundary or on the smaller area on which you are laying your grid, such as a bedside table, for example.
3. Place a crystal in each of the opposite corners of the room or space.
4. Link up the crystals with a crystal wand or the power of your mind.
5. When you're ready, dismantle the grid.

Grid-kit suggestions: Grounding, protective, and anchoring crystals; high-vibration light-bringing crystals; Shungite, Black Tourmaline, Carnelian, Mookaite Jasper, Polychrome Jasper, or Selenite

PENTAGRAM

ABUNDANCE AND ATTRACTION

A pentagram draws the assistance of the gods—archetypal, universal forces—from "above" to down "below," infusing earthly projects with creative and protective power. It has no innate connection to the dark side, contrary to what superstitious people may say. The upward point represents spirit, while the other four points represent the elements of earth, air, fire, and water, all of which are united in this form. It represents the descent of a spark of the divine into tangible matter.

Form: A pentagram is drawn with a continuous, flowing line in five straight strokes—in whichever direction feels most comfortable—creating a five-pointed star. The five spiked "arms" enclose a central "womb," creating a defensive, protective pentagon at the center. The pentagram can be placed into a circle to further strengthen the protection it offers.

Uses: The pentagram has long been believed to be a potent source of protection against evil, acting as a shield that defends the wearer, home, or environment from negative energy. It is also traditionally used to attract abundance and prosperity. An inverted pentagram is helpful for looking deep into oneself, or for transmuting toxic matter, because it draws an element and its properties—such as the cleansing and replenishing power of water—to where it is needed.

Timing: No special timing. If you are using it to attract abundance or when commencing a new project, lay the grid at a new moon or in the spring. Lay it on the summer solstice to bring fresh vitality into your life, or at the winter solstice to transmute toxic patterns and begin a new cycle.

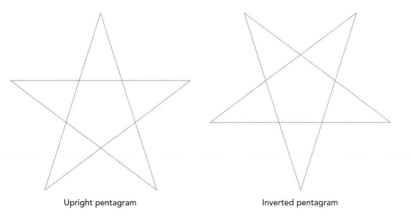

Upright pentagram   Inverted pentagram

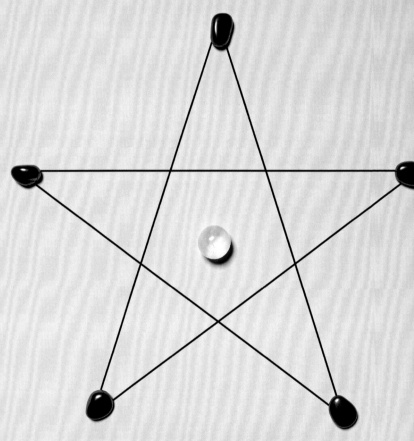

Smoky Quartz surrounds Selenite to cleanse
a space and draw in light.

YOU WILL NEED:

- Five appropriate crystals
- Keystone

TO LAY THE GRID:

1. Hold your cleansed crystals in your hands and state your intention for the grid.
2. Place the first crystal at the top point.
3. Follow the line down to place the second crystal at the bottom.
4. Place the third crystal up and across.
5. Place the fourth crystal straight across.
6. Place the fifth crystal down at the remaining bottom point.
7. Join up the crystals with the power of your mind, remembering to return to your starting point.
8. Lay your keystone in the center, stating your intention once more.
9. When you're ready, dismantle the grid.

Grid-kit suggestions: Grounding, protective, and anchoring crystals; cleansing crystals; high-vibration light-bringing crystals; abundance crystals

HEXAGRAM

PROTECTION AND CLEANSING

The hexagram is another ancient symbol of protection and of the unification of opposing forces. At the junction of heaven and earth, it balances the primary emotional energy of the universe—love. It reminds us that we are children of both spirit and earth. The hexagram's six points are said to stand for the six days of creation, and to represent the six attributes of God: power, wisdom, majesty, love, mercy, and justice.

Form: Two interlocked, overlapping equilateral triangles create a hexagram, but they can be extended to fill a space. A unicursal hexagram is drawn with a single line, and it is particularly useful for unification grids.

Uses: This grid balances internal and external needs and desires. The first triangle draws down light and then locks it into place, while the second triangle clears toxicity and grounds energy. It is an excellent symbol of protection. Place the name or photograph of a person who needs assistance into the center under the keystone, and the protective energy will be transmitted to them. Sitting within a hexagram can also clear mind chatter and help overcome insomnia, especially if the grid is created from Auralite 23 or Amethyst.

Timing: No special timing.

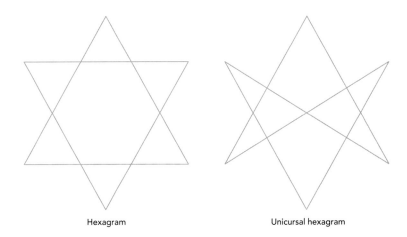

Hexagram   Unicursal hexagram

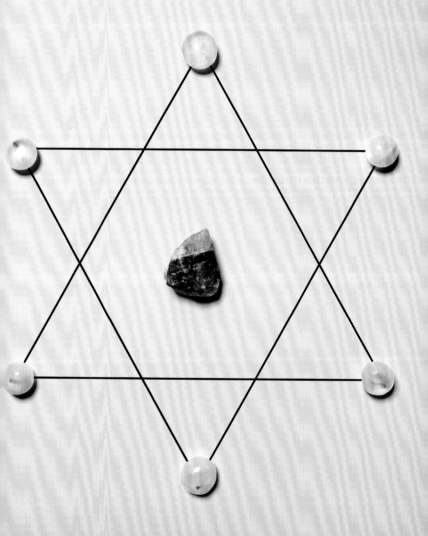

An Amethyst and Snow Quartz keystone surrounded by Selenite to
infuse light and mutual understanding into a neighborhood.

YOU WILL NEED:

- Three clearing crystals
- Three light-bringing crystals
- Keystone

TO LAY THE GRID:

1. Hold your crystals in your hands and state your intention for the grid.
2. Lay the first triangle, placing clearing crystals on each point.
3. Join up the points and spray the grid with clearing essence. (Dowse to see whether the triangle should point up or down.)
4. Lay the light-bringing crystals in an overlocking triangle over the top of the first. Join up the points, starting with the first crystal you laid.
5. Place your keystone in the center, stating your intention once more. When you're ready, dismantle the grid.

Grid-kit suggestions: Grounding, protective, and anchoring or cleansing crystals in the downward triangle. High-vibration, light-bringing crystals or abundance crystals in upward triangle.

SQUARE

BALANCING AND SOLIDIFYING

The square template is one of the most basic and versatile of grids. It anchors intention and grounds energy. In its simplest form, it is created by placing a crystal in the four corners of a room or at the four corners of a bed. But a square grid's power isn't limited to its perimeters. It creates an energetic cube, so it can be used to grid a building or another specific site. As a protective layout, the square grid consolidates energy, balancing and solidifying it. It also repels detrimental energies and so creates a contained safe space. The grid can be extended by placing anchoring crystals outside the square, which holds grid energy in place for long periods of time and is particularly useful for gridding a house.

Form: A square has four equal sides and four equal angles. However, this template can be adapted to fit the shape of a space. It can be extended on two sides to become a rectangle or slanted to create a parallelogram. Not all the square's sides and angles have to remain equal for the energetic effect to become apparent.

Uses: A square layout protects a space from geopathic stress or electromagnetic pollution, and it also creates a safe space in which to live, work, or meditate. Place it around your bed if you have trouble sleeping, or around a room to calm the atmosphere and reduce noise levels—or, place it on and around your head to create clarity. The square is also used in situations where limits need to be defined, or where out-of-control energy needs to be contained. Finally, squares are excellent for aligning goals and building community.

Timing: No special timing.

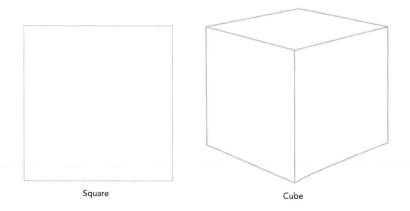

Square

Cube

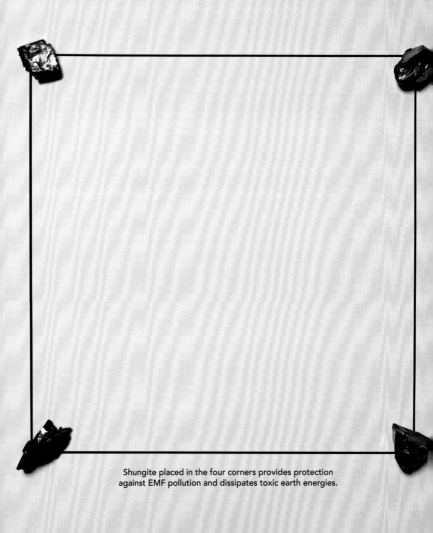

Shungite placed in the four corners provides protection against EMF pollution and dissipates toxic earth energies.

Rectangle and
parallelograms

YOU WILL NEED:

- Four crystals of similar type and size
- Keystone

TO LAY THE GRID:

1. Hold your crystals in your hands and state your intention for the grid.
2. Lay your first crystal in one corner. (Dowse to see which crystal should be the first one laid.)
3. Lay your second crystal in the corner to the right of the first.
4. Lay your third crystal below that in the next corner.
5. Lay your final crystal in the last corner.
6. Join up the corners and the crystals with a wand or the power of your mind. Feel the energy pinging around the grid as you do so, lighting it up.
7. If appropriate, lay a keystone as close to the center as possible to anchor the energy. The activation is now complete.
8. Leave the grid in place for as long as necessary. This is a long-term protection grid, so you may leave it in place for many months. Cleanse as often as necessary.
9. When you're ready, dismantle the grid.

Grid-kit suggestions: Grounding, protective, anchoring, or cleansing crystals.
Shungite with Herkimer Diamond is especially appropriate for this grid if your intention is to protect against electric and magnetic fields.

ZIGZAG

ENVIRONMENTAL CLEANSING

A zigzag structure is inherently more stable than a straight line; it can better absorb stresses, maintaining its high-energy output. It is ideal for laying around or within a building to create protection and to discharge static or electromagnetic smog.

Form: A line of crystals is laid along a boundary wall from one end to the other in a zigzag fashion. To protect or clear the space, another line is laid along the opposite wall. (This double line is more powerful than a single one because it contains the energy within the space being encompassed.) The crystals can be alternated. Place clearing crystals on the top edge of the zig and light-bringing crystals on the zag.

Uses: The zigzag layout is particularly useful for healing sick-building syndrome and neutralizing environmental pollution. It is also helpful if you want to clear clutter or energetically declutter a space.

Timing: No special timing.

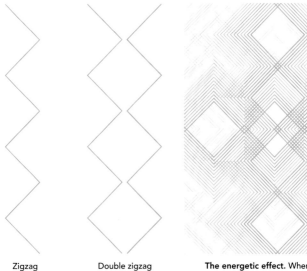

Zigzag   Double zigzag

The energetic effect. When a double zigzag is laid, the energy moves toward the center of the grid to fill the whole area with protective, transmuting energy.

Smoky Quartz and
Selenite are an ideal
combination for healing
sick-building syndrome.

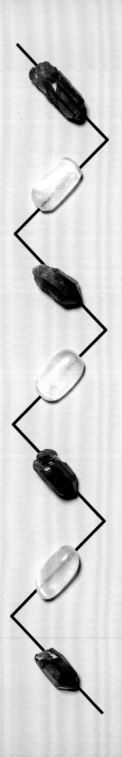

YOU WILL NEED:

- Sufficient crystals to run the length of the wall at regular intervals, depending on the length of the wall
- An anchor stone can be placed at each end

TO LAY THE GRID:

1. Hold your crystals in your hands and state your intention for the grid.
2. Lay the first crystal against the left-hand wall. Begin with an anchor stone, if appropriate. (Use your intuition to decide.)
3. Lay a zigzag all the way to the right-hand wall. Place an anchor stone at the end if this is appropriate.
4. If creating the double zigzag, move to the opposite wall and repeat the operation.
5. Join up the crystals with a crystal wand or the power of your mind. (If making a double zigzag, walk from one end to the other, and then back to the starting point.)
6. When you're ready, dismantle the grid.

Grid-kit suggestions: Black Tourmaline, Shungite, Smoky Quartz, Herkimer Diamond, Selenite, Quartz

SPIRAL

VORTEX ENERGY MANAGEMENT

A spiral creates vortex energy—that is, a whirling mass of energy generated from a central point and either radiated outward or sucked inward, depending on its electrostatic charge—and is a basis for accelerating growth and switching on positive DNA potential. Depending on which way it is placed, a spiral draws energy down into its center—a crystal placed at the top begins the process—or radiates energy from a crystal placed at its center. So, when you're joining the crystals with your wand or the power of your mind, do not go back to the first crystal you laid. Instead, depending on your intention, spiral the energy out and away or down into the spiral's center. You can also use a multi-armed spiral when you want to radiate transmuting and re-energizing vibrations out into the surrounding area for as great a distance as possible.

Form: You could lay a "perfect logarithmic spiral" using the Golden Ratio, but this is not essential for grid work. Instead, dowse or use your intuition to check whether you should be using a clockwise or counterclockwise spiral and how many crystals are needed for your grid.

Uses: A spiral re-energizes a space or helps to begin a project, sending the idea out into the universe ahead of you. Use it also to irradiate a "dead" or empty space with crystal energy, especially after energetic clearing has taken place. This is a particularly useful grid for map or photographic work.

Timing: Lay a spiral grid at any time. However, a drawing-down or inward grid is particularly potent at new moon, and a radiating one is most powerful at full moon.

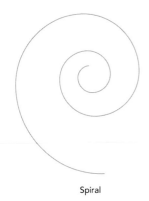

Spiral

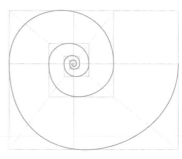

Golden Ratio spiral

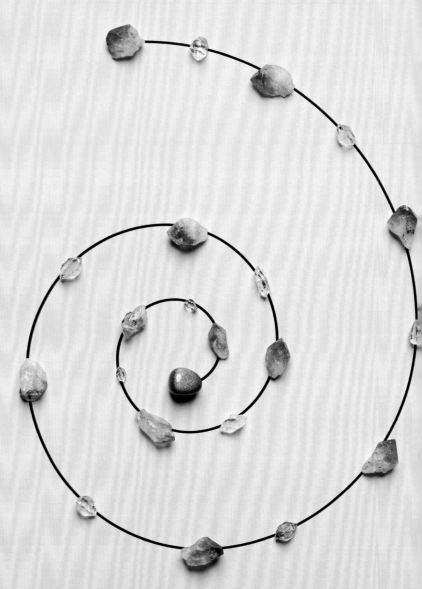

Citrine and Herkimer Diamonds radiate the energy from a Gold-stone keystone into the environment.

YOU WILL NEED:

- Sufficient crystals to outline the spiral.
- Keystone

TO LAY THE GRID:

1. Create your spiral. (String is ideal for creating the form.)
2. Hold your crystals in your hands and state your intention for the grid.
3. Place the first crystal (the keystone) at the center or at the end, depending on your intention. (If you're drawing in energy, you'll lay the outer stone first; if you're radiating it, lay the center stone first.)
4. Complete the spiral, laying crystals along it at intervals.
5. Join up the spiral with the power of your mind or a crystal wand, remembering not to return to your starting point. If you began at the center, draw the wand out and away. If you began at the outer edge, tap the wand firmly at the center and then place the keystone there.
6. When you're ready, dismantle the grid.

Grid-kit suggestions: Citrine, Herkimer Diamond, Selenite, Sunstone, Goldstone, Smoky Quartz

SUNBURST

ENERGIZING AND REVITALIZING

A sunburst layout is highly energizing, and it radiates its energy over a large area, so it is particularly suited to placement on the ground or over a map. Although it's typical to start laying crystals in the center of the sunburst and to work outward from there, it can be helpful to dowse or use your intuition for the placements of crystals before you begin. This is because a directional alignment—that is, one that's aligned to the points of the compass—may need to be set out first, and the central stone could be laid first or last according to whether the crystals are placed to draw energy in or out. The layout can always be adjusted later to fine-tune the energies.

Unlike many other grids, this layout is not activated by joining with a wand, as the intention is to radiate the energy as widely as possible. Instead, a radiating sunburst is set in motion by the intention of your mind. When you're placing the crystals, remember that points channel energy in the direction in which they face. If a point is facing toward you or to a specific spot, it channels energy into you or to that spot. If it's pointing away from you, it sends energy outward.

Form: A sunburst grid can have short or long arms, and they may be equal, unequal, or a mixture of both. Crystals can be laid in lines or simply placed at each end around a central keystone. It can be as large or as small as you wish. If you're building a large sunburst to remain in place over time, use large raw crystals and ensure that they can be cleansed and energized as appropriate. Or, soak them in Petaltone Z14 if you intend to bury them in the ground. (Always be sure to mark where such a grid lies.)

Uses: First and foremost, sunburst grids are energizing grids. But they can have other functions, too. A sunburst can be built of detoxifying crystals, offering ongoing cleansing and protection to an area that's particularly polluted, for example. It can also be used to direct energy away from a particular space by placing protective crystals pointing toward the center on the side that needs shielding and by placing radiating crystals pointing away from the center on the opposite side. And, finally, a radiating sunburst can send healing over huge distances to a specific recipient.

Timing: Lay a sunburst grid at any time. However, it is particularly potent in the spring for energizing, and before winter for detoxifying.

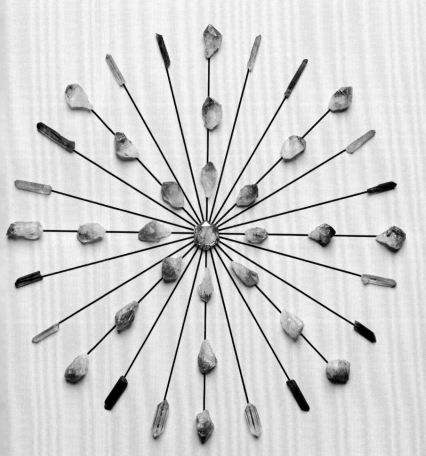

Citrine and Smoky Quartz radiate the vibrant energy of a Tangerine
Sun Aura Quartz into the environment.

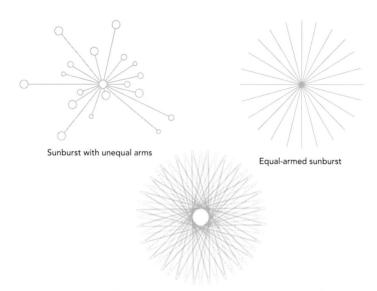

Sunburst with unequal arms

Equal-armed sunburst

Energetic effect. A sunburst grid doesn't just emit straight lines of energy; it also creates an interlocking energy grid that either radiates or draws in energy, according to the direction in which the crystals face.

YOU WILL NEED:

- Sufficient crystals for your purpose (Dowse before beginning to determine exactly how many and which kind.)

TO LAY THE GRID:

1. Hold your crystals in your hands. State your intention for the grid.
2. Dowse or use your intuition for the appropriate positions for your cleansed crystals and lay them roughly in a sunburst shape. You don't necessarily need to lay the central keystone first. Trust your intuition to tell you when to place it in your grid.
3. Stand at the center of the grid (or focus your attention into its center) and state your intention.
4. Fine-tune the grid by aligning crystals carefully or allowing them to roll into the position they choose.
5. Check that the final placements are effective by dowsing or using your intuition.
6. Activate the grid with a crystal wand or the power of your mind.
7. When you're ready, dismantle the grid.

Grid-kit suggestions: Carnelian, Celtic Quartz, Citrine, Quartz, Red Jasper, Sunstone, Smoky Quartz, Shungite, Flint, Hematite

THE BODY

HEALING AND REBALANCING

Your body itself is a grid. Crystals can be placed on the chakras to cleanse and rebalance them, and they can be placed on and around the body—and over specific organs—to restore well-being. For example, when laid around the head, crystals such as Auralite 23 are particularly effective for shutting off mind chatter to create a quiet headspace and to reduce stress. This can also help to overcome insomnia. Crystals placed over the kidneys and adrenals switch off the fight-or-flight response.

Form: Appropriate crystals can be laid on the body as required. The Tree of Life grid (page 88), for instance, is particularly effective when laid over the body. Even though it is one of the most potent physical grids, it is also one of the simplest. It requires only one stone over the higher heart chakra to stimulate the immune system, and one grounding stone, such as Flint or Smoky Quartz, at the feet. Use Bloodstone, Quantum Quattro, or a dowsed stone.

Timing: Lay a grid whenever necessary or at new moon for a thorough chakra cleanse and recharge.

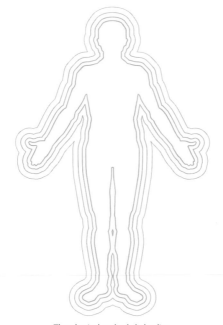

The physical and subtle bodies

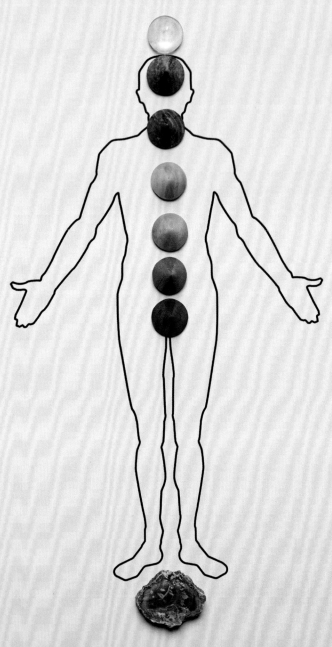

Petrified Wood on the Earth star chakra anchors a Red Jasper, Orange Carnelian, Yellow Jasper, Green Aventurine, Sodalite, Lapis Lazuli, and Clear Quartz chakra cleanse and balance layout.

YOU WILL NEED:

- Appropriate chakra or healing crystals

TO LAY THE GRID:

1. Choose a place and time when you will not be disturbed. Be sure to switch off your mobile phone.
2. Hold your crystals in your hands and state your intention for the grid.
3. Lie down and cover yourself with a blanket, if necessary, so that you are warm and comfortable.
4. To lay a grid on or around a physical body, dowse or intuit where each crystal should go, and choose crystals by the same method. You could, for instance, place an appropriate crystal on each chakra. You can also lay a crystal directly over an organ or position the crystal over a specific place, such as the throat. Additionally, you can place the crystals around your head to shut off mind chatter and overcome insomnia. If you are laying the grid on yourself, start with your feet and work upward. Ensure that you have placed a grounding and transmuting crystal below your feet.
5. Leave the grid in place for ten to twenty minutes.
6. Gather up the crystals in the reverse order in which you placed them. Dismantle the grid.

Grid-kit suggestions: Flint, Smoky Quartz, Red Jasper, Carnelian, Yellow Calcite, Green Aventurine, Blue Lace Agate, Lapis Lazuli, Quartz, Blue Kyanite, Polychrome Jasper, Mookaite Jasper, Shungite, Quantum Quattro, Bloodstone, Que Sera.

CHAPTER FOUR

ADVANCED GRIDS

THE GRIDS IN THIS SECTION may look complicated, but they are just as easy to set out as the basic grids in the previous chapter. Simply follow the templates. Some complex grids create very powerful energetic patterns and are more suitable for use by experienced crystal workers. Such grids may require careful dismantling when their task is complete, as the energetic imprint of these grids lasts much longer because of the complex geometry involved in the energetic net. Other grids can be left in the ether (energetic space) to naturally dissipate once the crystals have been removed. It all depends on the purpose for which they have been laid. If a grid has been laid to resolve a specific confrontation, for instance, once that conflict is over, the grid needs to be energetically dismantled. But if the grid is to instill long-lasting peace into an environment or ongoing situation, it can be left to dissipate naturally once the crystals have been removed.

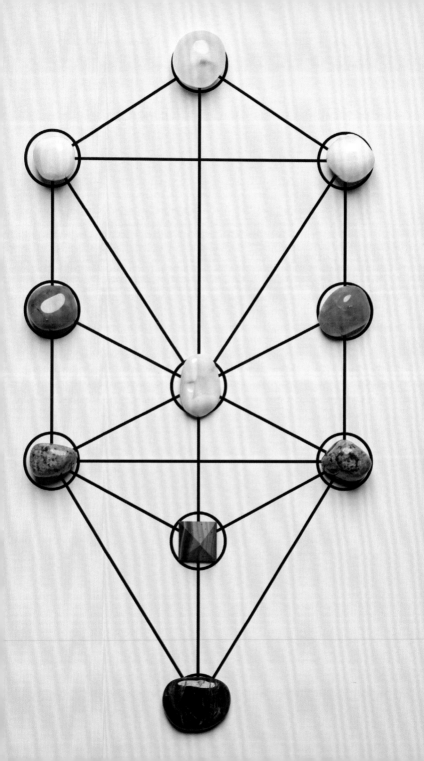

FLOWER OF LIFE

THE FOUNDATION OF CREATION

The Flower of Life has been regarded as a symbol of self-knowledge—and knowledge of the universe as a whole—for thousands of years. For this grid, precise placement of crystals is necessary to control the flow of energy along the pathways.

Form: The Flower of Life grows from the Vesica Piscis through six-fold symmetry, which means that the pattern replicates itself equally around its central point with six axes that remain constant, regardless of how many times the grid is expanded. The pattern is the same when viewed from all angles, and the energetic effect is three dimensional. The center of each circle is located on the circumference of one of the surrounding circles. Many other grid shapes lie within the Flower, too. The Seed of Life lies at its heart. Its seven overlapping circles create a flower-like pattern. An outer circle forms a protective barrier to negativity and invasion by outside forces, while the inner circle represents conception. Six cells cluster around the central core to create new life, a feature also found in the Fruit of Life grid.

Uses: The Flower of Life and the Seed of Life are particularly potent for manifestation grids that bring goals and desires to a successful conclusion, or for a protective grid to enhance the energies within an area. The grid can also be used to balance the chakras of the physical body and the energy vortex points within the immediate or wider environment for earth healing. It is also a useful focus for meditation and for sending distant healing to other parts of the world either for an individual's needs or for public situations such as war, famine, or natural disasters.

Timing: This grid can be laid any time, but it can be extremely effective when laid under the full moon. The Seed of Life is particularly potent when it's set out at a new moon or in the spring.

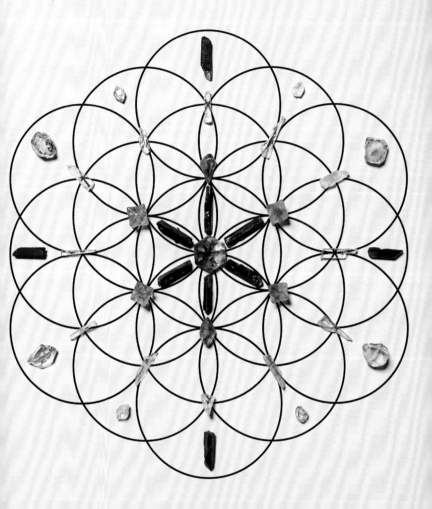

Amethyst, Danburite, Herkimer Diamond, and Smoky Quartz radiate calming energy and universal love out into the environment in Flower of Life.

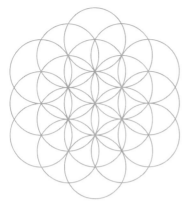

Unboundaried Flower of Life

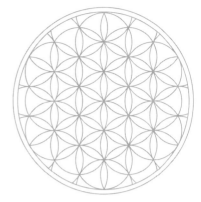

Boundaried Flower of Life

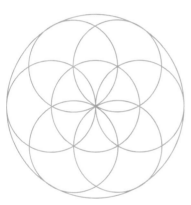

The Seed of Life

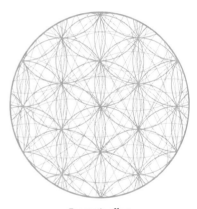

Energetic effect.
The Flower of Life replicates and radiates harmonious energy equally in all directions, but the flow can be controlled by the crystal pattern superimposed on it, according to the intention of the grid.

YOU WILL NEED:

- Template
- Cleansed and empowered crystals according to the grid shape you wish to lay within the Flower
- Sufficient crystals for the outer circle, if creating a boundaried grid
- Keystone

TO LAY THE GRID:

1. If you are laying the complete Flower of Life or the Seed of Life inner grid, you will need a template to follow, because precise positioning is important. Lay the template on a colored background or a material appropriate for your purpose.
2. Hold your crystals in your hands and state your intention for the grid.
3. Place the keystone in the center of the grid to anchor it.
4. With focused attention, lay a crystal in the center of each flower shape.
5. Lay crystals radiating along the petals of each flower or along the arcs, according to what pleases your inner eye. Trust your intuition.
6. Lay the outer circle with protective crystals, if you're creating a boundaried grid.
7. To activate the grid, gaze at it through softly focused eyes until the energy lights up the grid. (If you're not an experienced practitioner, this may be something you sense or intuit rather than see with your physical eyes.)
8. To dismantle the grid, remove the keystone, and then remove the crystals in the reverse order in which you laid them. The space in which the grid was laid will almost certainly require sound or a clearing essence to completely dismantle it since its energetic imprint is long-lasting.

Grid-kit suggestions: Chakra crystals, Quartz, Herkimer Diamond, Rose Quartz, Rhodochrosite, Smoky Quartz, Blue Kyanite, Imperial Topaz, Rhodozite

TREE OF LIFE

THE NATURE OF THE DIVINE

The Tree of Life is used in Kabala to understand the nature of the divine and the way in which the world was created. Depicting the descent of spirit into matter, it is regarded by practitioners as a "map of reality," each of thirty-two pathways leading to an expansion of the knowledge of the divine or the wisdom of the universal mind. In certain approaches, it is the path to knowing God or the Eternal; in others, it is the path to knowing the Self. The Celtic Tree of Life is drawn with the branches reaching skyward and the roots spreading into the earth below. The branches and roots link in a circle, symbolizing the Druidic belief in the connection between heaven and earth and the eternal nature of cyclic life and afterlife.

Form: The Tree of Life arises from of the center of the Flower of Life. Or, in the Celtic approach, it is drawn as a tree with the roots placed deep in the Earth and the branches reaching up to heaven, united by the tree's trunk. In some Celtic forms, the branches and the roots also meet. The Tree of Life can be stretched and expanded to cover the human body or an area within the environment.

Uses: In gridwork, crystals are placed on ten major points of the Kabalistic Tree to bring about integration, since the Tree of Life is used for grids that balance heaven and earth or that lead to a deeper spiritual understanding. The Kabalistic Tree of Life is particularly useful for laying on and around the body to balance the chakras and energy flow around the body. It can also be buried or laid in the external environment, where it can be left in place for long periods of time. The Celtic Tree of Life is the perfect grid for placing in the home to heal the ancestral line and for taking forgiveness back into the past—but it requires a cloth or baseplate on which the tree is printed to place the crystals to maximize effect.

Timing: The Tree of Life can be laid at any time, but the Celtic Tree is particularly effective when adjusted to the cycles and seasons of the year by changing the crystals at the solstices and equinoxes.

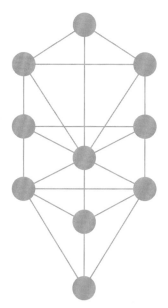

Kabalistic Tree of Life

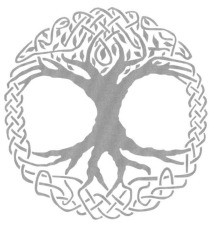

Celtic Tree of Life

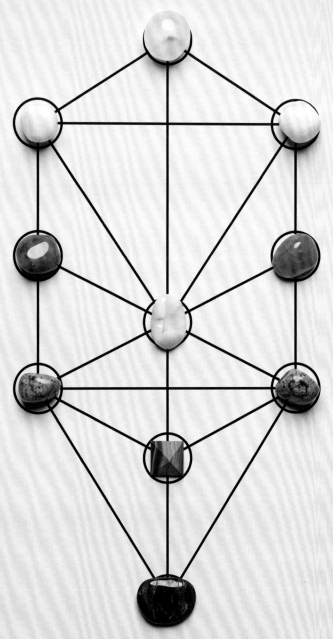

A polished Shungite anchor stone below a Malachite pyramid,
African Turquoises, Blue Lace Agate keystone, Orange Carnelians,
Rose Quartzes, and Selenite light-bringer cleanse the chakras and
enhance the flow of spiritual energy around the body.

YOU WILL NEED:

- Appropriate template and background
- Keystone and anchor stones

For the Kabalistic Tree: Ten appropriate crystals

For the Celtic Tree: A selection of light-bringing, grounding, and detoxifying crystals

TO LAY THE GRID:

1. Select your template and background color according to your intention.
2. Hold your crystals in your hands and state your intention for the grid.
3. If you are laying the Kabalistic Tree to expand your awareness, begin by placing an anchor stone at the base, and then work your way up the tree, using appropriate crystals. Place your anchor stone at the central point of the grid (three circles up from the base).
4. If you are laying the Kabalistic Tree to draw divine energy down into matter, begin by placing the keystone at the topmost circle and then proceed down to the base, where you'll lay the anchor stone.
5. Join the crystals with a crystal wand or the power of your mind.
6. To dismantle the grid, remove the keystone, and then remove the crystals in the reverse order in which you laid them. The space in which the grid was laid will almost certainly require sound or a clearing essence to completely dismantle it since its energetic imprint is long-lasting.

Grid-kit suggestions: Ancestralite, Kambaba Jasper, Celtic Quartz, Cradle of Life (Humankind), Freedom Stone, Hematite, Dumortierite, Anandalite™, Selenite, Yellow Calcite, Green Calcite, Clear Calcite

CHAPTER FIVE

SPECIFIC GRIDS

THE SPECIFIC EXAMPLE GRIDS included in this section are intended to inspire you to begin your own grid creation. You can adapt the crystals within the grids to suit your own individual needs or adapt the grid templates themselves in accordance with your intuition.

Dowse or use your intuition to find which crystals are appropriate, especially when you're creating mood-altering grids. You'll find suggestions for this in the grid-kits, but please don't limit yourself to these. Be creative and inspired!

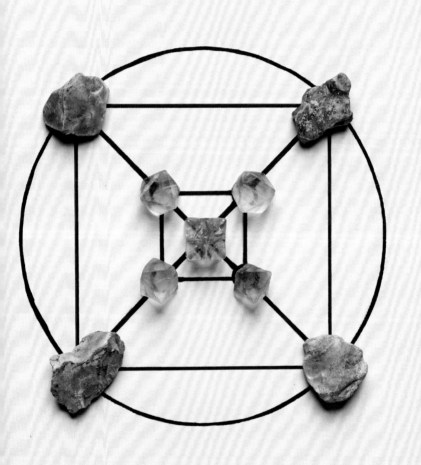

GROUNDING

Many people find it difficult to anchor themselves on the planet. Impractical and disconnected, they "live in their heads," so to speak. But this grid can help. Grounding guides you to settle yourself in the present moment and to actualize your intentions.

Using the grid: This grid is best laid directly onto and around your body while you are lying on the floor, or in the environment. But you can also lay it beneath your bed to anchor you while you sleep.

Timing: This grid can be used at any time. It is particularly important before and after carrying out rituals that connect you to angels and higher beings. It is also helpful before any kind of spiritual opening-up, meditation, visualization, or even a ritual that doesn't involve crystal grids, as it keeps your energy grounded.

Color and background: Earthy colors such as brown, ochre, or green, or natural materials.

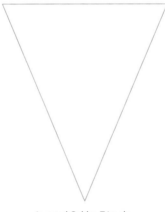

Inverted Golden Triangle

YOU WILL NEED:

- Three grounding crystals
- Two Magnesite
- Two Charoite or Flint

TO LAY THE GRID:

1. Hold your cleansed crystals in your hands and state your intention.
2. Lie down comfortably to get a sense of the space required.
3. Sit up again and place a Smoky Quartz or other grounding crystal below your feet.
4. Place a Charoite or Flint on each knee.
5. Lie down and place a Magnesite on each side of your body in the groin crease.
6. Place a Flint, Smoky Quartz, or other grounding crystal on either side of you, level with your navel.
7. Place your hands on the Magnesite.
8. Use the power of your mind to connect the triangle.
9. With your mind, feel the grid connecting to the Earth star chakra beneath your feet and then to the Gaia gateway chakra and the planet below.
10. Lie still for fifteen minutes, enjoying this connection to Mother Earth.
11. Remove the crystals in the opposite order in which you placed them, placing at least one in your pocket to remind yourself of your experience. Choose whichever crystal resonates with you and carry it in your pocket for as long as you feel connected to it. When you feel that the crystal has lost its charge, you can repeat the layout.

Grid-kit suggestions: Brown Carnelian, Charoite, Flint, Hematite, Magnesite, Smoky Quartz, Mookaite Jasper, Polychrome Jasper

GENERAL WELL-BEING

The upper and lower loops on a lemniscate layout do not need to be of equal size, and they can be adjusted to fit your body as required. This well-being layout connects your thymus (higher heart chakra), which controls your immune system, with your extended energy body, toning up your overall integrated holistic energy system—that is, your physical, emotional, mental, and spiritual selves—to ensure well-being.

Using the grid: This grid is particularly useful if you suspect you're coming down with a cold or the flu, but use it at any time to support your well-being.

Timing: Use whenever you feel in need of a tone-up of your physical or subtle energies.

Color and background: Blue is a traditional healing color.

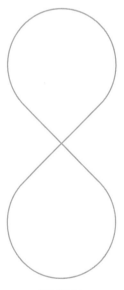

Lemniscate

Selenite above the head, Bloodstone over the thymus, and an anchor stone at the feet complete the simple lemniscate layout.

YOU WILL NEED:

- Clearing crystal
- Light-bringing crystal
- Immune-balancing crystal

TO LAY THE GRID:

1. Hold your crystals in your hands and state your intention for the grid.
2. Lie down.
3. Place a clearing crystal beneath your feet (sit up to do so).
4. Place a light-bringing crystal above your head.
5. Place an immune-balancing crystal halfway up your breastbone over the higher heart chakra.
6. Use the power of your mind to connect the lemniscate over and around you.
7. Remain in the grid for five to fifteen minutes, focusing your attention and breathing gently into the immune-balancing crystal. If you become aware of energy that needs to shift out of your body, send it down to the crystal at your feet for transmutation.
8. Remove the crystals in the reverse order in which you laid them, then cleanse them.

Note: The grid can also be laid beneath your bed.

Grid-kit suggestions: *Immune-balancing crystals:* Bloodstone; Green Aventurine; Que Sera (Llanoite); Quantum Quattro; Cherry, Rose, Smoky, or Emerald Quartz

EMF CLEARING

If you're sensitive to them, electromagnetic fields (EMFs) may have a detrimental effect on your health, so regularly clearing your energy body is both sensible and simple. EMFs are generated by computers, WiFi, cell phones, power lines, electricity-generating stations, "smart-meters," and electrical equipment in general. EMFs make a significant contribution to sick-building syndrome.

Using the grid: If you suffer from general malaise and ongoing tiredness, if you feel worse in a particular environment and better when away from it, or if you use your cell phone or computer regularly, spend five minutes in the grid each evening to clear your energy field.

Timing: Daily, or as necessary.

Background and color: Natural materials, such as wood or slate, work well for this grid.

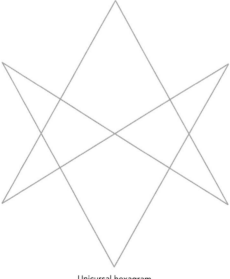

Unicursal hexagram

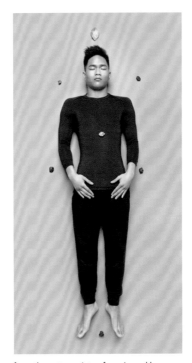

Black Tourmalines form the outer points of a unicursal hexagram around the body with Herkimer Diamond light-bringers over the head and on the chest.

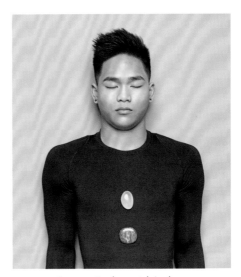

Immune stimular crystals in place.

YOU WILL NEED:

• Light-bringing crystal: Selenite, Amethyst, Herkimer Diamond, or Rose Quartz
• Five EMF-clearing crystals
• Herkimer Diamond or other keystone

TO LAY THE GRID:

1. Hold your crystals in your hands and state your intention for the grid.
2. Lie down comfortably on a bed or the floor.
3. Place a light-bringing crystal over your head.
4. Place an EMF-clearing crystal to your right-hand side, level with your groin.
5. Place an EMF-clearing crystal level with your left ear.
6. Place an EMF-clearing crystal below your feet.
7. Place an EMF-clearing crystal level with your right ear.
8. Place an EMF-clearing crystal on your left-hand side, level with your groin.
9. Place a Herkimer Diamond or other keystone over your higher heart chakra (thymus).
10. Use the power of your mind to activate the grid.
11. Breathe out, consciously allowing the EMF energy to drain down toward the crystal at your feet.
12. Breathe into your belly, drawing energy from the light-bringing crystal down through the grid and into your energy body.
13. Repeat the breaths ten times and lie within the grid for as long as you feel you need to. Trust your intuition to tell you when to get up.
14. Remove the crystals in the reverse order in which they were laid, then cleanse them. Unless you live close to a source of EMFs, place crystals in the sun and air to recharge.

Grid-kit suggestions: *EMF-clearing crystals:* Amber, Shungite, Black Tourmaline, Herkimer Diamond, Smoky Quartz, Lepidolite, Green Aventurine, Amethyst, Amber, Cherry and Emerald Quartz, Rose Quartz, Celtic Quartz, Ajoite in Shattukite, Amazonite, Lepidolite.

SUNSHINE SUPER CRYSTALS

THE S.A.D. ANTIDOTE

Many people suffer from "the winter blues," or seasonal affective disorder (S.A.D.), due to a lack of sunlight, but using appropriate sunshine crystals and a layout based on the hexagram can help to counteract that effect. This grid can be laid on and around your body to energetically stimulate the pituitary gland and boost hormone production, or it can be placed in your environment in order to infuse it with solar power. Placing the crystals in the sun for a week or two before the autumnal equinox charges them up and stores the sunlight in the crystals so that they're ready for the coming winter.

Using the grid: Use the grid for a few minutes daily whenever you find yourself feeling S.A.D. or lay it under your bed. This works especially well during the winter months, but it also helps to boost low moods year-round.

Timing: As a preventative measure, start laying the grid at the autumnal equinox around September 22, and continue until the vernal (spring) equinox on March 20. (Switch the dates around if you live in the southern hemisphere.)

Color and background: Golden or yellow cloth.

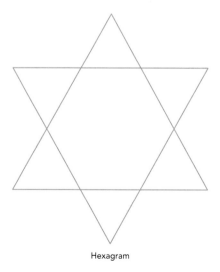

Hexagram

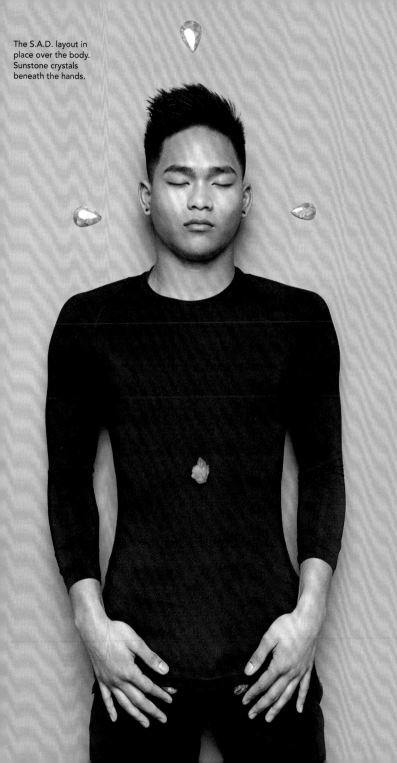

The S.A.D. layout in place over the body. Sunstone crystals beneath the hands.

YOU WILL NEED:

- Clearing crystal such as Shungite, Flint, or Smoky Quartz
- Five sunshine crystals
- Small sunshine keystone

TO LAY THE GRID:

1. Begin by placing the cleansed crystals in the sunshine for one or two weeks prior to the equinox.
2. Hold the crystals in your hands and state your intention for the grid.
3. Place a clearing crystal point-down below your feet or at the base of the layout.
4. Place one sunshine crystal point-down above your head or at the top of the grid.
5. Place a sunshine crystal on either side of your head, level with the bottom of your ears; or on either side of the layout, pointing inward.
6. Hold two sunshine crystals over your groin creases or place them below the previous two crystals in the layout, pointing inward.
7. Place a small sunshine keystone crystal over your solar plexus or in the center of the layout and restate your intention.
8. Lie quietly for ten to twenty minutes, breathing into your solar plexus and absorbing the crystal energies.
9. When you're ready to stand up, remove the crystals in the reverse order in which they were laid, then cleanse them. Or, leave the grid under your bed.
10. Place the keystone in your pocket, where you'll feel its energies radiating into your body, and keep it there for as long as you feel connected to it (be sure to cleanse it regularly). When you feel that the crystal has lost its charge, you can repeat the layout after recharging the crystals in sunlight, with a purpose-made essence, or on a large Carnelian first.
11. Place the crystals outside to recharge whenever there is sufficient sunshine.

Grid-kit suggestions: Citrine, Sunstone, Yellow Calcite, Golden Healer Quartz, Celtic Quartz, Quartz, Rutilated Quartz, Tiger's Eye, Orange Kyanite, Carnelian, Golden Azeztulite, Rainbow Mayanite, Mookaite Jasper, Bumble Bee Jasper, Yellow Opal, Yellow Jasper, Zincite

SUPPORT DURING SERIOUS ILLNESS

The Merkaba is an excellent resource if you or someone you know is moving through a serious or chronic illness. It's ideal for emotional and energetic support, and it sends constant healing vibes to the person in need. You might choose a center keystone that's especially suitable for the specific illness, or you might select one that will create centeredness and stability regardless of the condition. Either one works well.

Using the grid: Lay the grid in a place where it will not be disturbed. Under a bed is ideal if it is for your own illness. If not, place it over a photograph of the person.

Timing: Lay the grid as soon as it is needed and leave in place for the duration of the illness. Cleanse it regularly.

Color and background: Blue is the traditional color for healing.

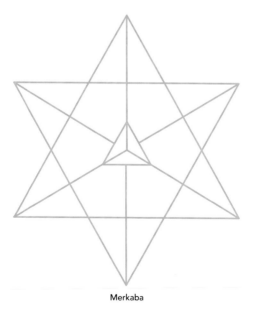

Merkaba

YOU WILL NEED:

- Appropriate crystals from the grid-kit
- Keystone
- Photograph of the person if they are not present

TO LAY THE GRID:

1. Hold your crystals in your hands and state your intention for the grid.
2. Choose a location where the grid can remain undisturbed.
3. Place the grid over a photograph or the name of the person who needs the support, or place it under your bed or over your own body.
4. Place an appropriate crystal on each of the six outer points.
5. Join each of the triangles with the power of your mind or a crystal wand.
6. Connect each outer crystal to the central keystone to link the crystals' power.
7. Leave the grid in place for as long as necessary. (If you're lying down with the grid on or around your body, lie in place for ten to twenty minutes, or longer.)
8. Remove the crystals in the reverse order in which they were laid, and cleanse them. (For extra cleansing, bury robust crystals in the ground after use, and leave delicate crystals in brown rice for an extra day or two.)

Grid-kit suggestions: Eye of the Storm (Judy's Jasper), Shungite, Flint, Jade, Quantum Quattro, Que Sera (Llanoite), Rose Quartz Cancer support: Klinoptilolith, Smoky Quartz, Rose Quartz, Quartz, Green Ridge Quartz, "Gunky" Golden Healer Quartz, Green Calcite Neuromuscular conditions: Natrolite and Scolecite, Rhodonite, Red Jasper, Fluorite, Dendritic Agate.

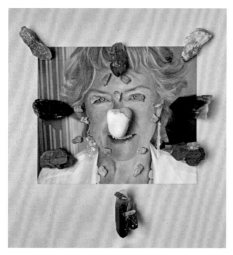

Klinoptilolith is the central keystone in this Smoky Quartz and Gunky Green Ridge hexagram to support during cancer treatment. Green Calcite has been added to soothe nausea and Celtic Golden Healer for overall well-being.

MENTAL CLARITY

Mental confusion can arise for a variety of reasons, some of which may require the laying of another grid to heal underlying causes. But clarity can also be obtained by focusing on a simple, expanded square grid. This is particularly useful when you are preparing to sit for an exam, before a job interview, or whenever you need to express yourself clearly. Place an appropriate stone, such as Apophyllite or Fluorite, as the keystone.

Using the grid: Place the grid in your environment or under the head of your bed where it will not be disturbed. Or, lie in the grid, with the top of your head just below the keystone or with the keystone placed on your forehead, if a friend or partner can lay the grid around you.

Timing: No specific timing.

Color and background: Yellow is the traditional color for mental clarity.

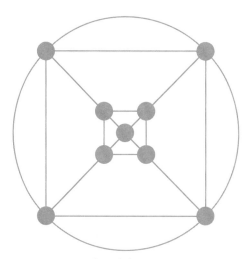

Expanded square

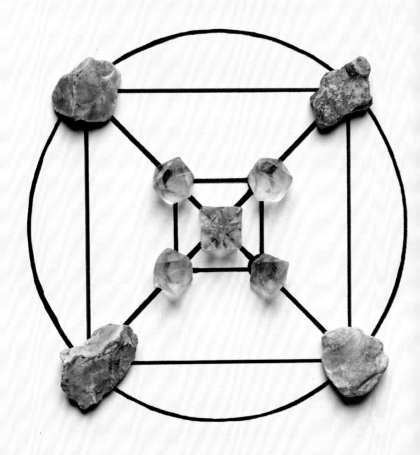

An Amethyst Merkaba forms the central focus of this simple
Fluorite and Flint mental clarity grid.

YOU WILL NEED:

- Four mental clarity crystals
- Four anchor crystals
- Crystals for the perimeter, if appropriate
- Keystone

TO LAY THE GRID:

1. Hold your crystals in your hands and state your intention for the grid.
2. Place the four mental clarity crystals on the corners of the inner square.
   (If you are going to lie in the grid, make the square large enough so that you can comfortably lie down in it.)
3. Place the four anchor crystals on the corners of the outer square.
4. If appropriate, place crystals around the perimeter. (Dowse to ascertain if required.)
5. If you're going to be lying in the grid, lie down now.
6. Place the keystone in the center of the grid or on your forehead.
7. Use the power of your mind to connect the crystals, moving from the keystone out to the perimeter. Then trace the circle. Move back into the center of the grid and then out again to connect the outer square, then the inner one.
8. If you're laying the grid in your environment, leave it in place as long as you like.
   As long as you cleanse it regularly, you can leave it in place permanently.
   Or, if you're lying within the grid, do so for ten to twenty minutes, or longer, if it feels right to you.
9. When you're ready to dismantle the grid, remove the crystals in the reverse order in which they were laid, then cleanse them.

Grid-kit suggestions: Apophyllite, Fluorite, Auralite 23, Blue Lace Agate, Clear Quartz, Emerald, Dumortierite, Rhomboid Selenite, Azurite, anchor crystals.

CREATIVITY AND FERTILITY

The Seed of Life is the central core of the Flower of Life. It is the fundamental point of new beginnings and conception. This grid is perfect for facilitating both the inception of a new project and physical conception.

Using the grid: Lay this grid whenever you are starting a new project, or if you are hoping to conceive a magical or physical child. It can be helpful for inner child work, too.

Timing: Traditionally, a new moon, new year, or spring are the most auspicious times to begin new projects. Avoid the period preceding the winter solstice, as the life force is dormant then—but the period just after the winter solstice is an excellent time for physical conception. Or, lay the grid whenever you conceive a project and tend it carefully.

Color and background: The colors of blood and spring are appropriate backgrounds.

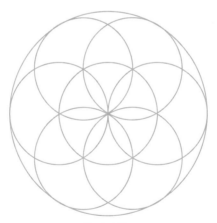

Seed of Life

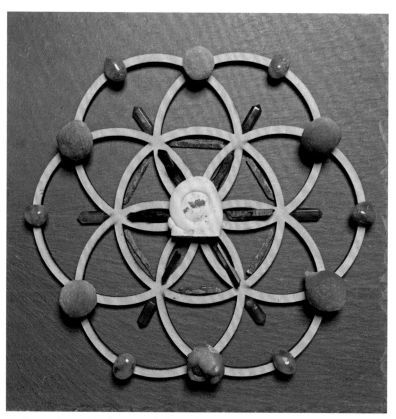

The womb-stone Menalite surrounded by six cleansing Smoky Quartz points forms the focus for a creativity and conception grid using Orange Kyanite, Orange Carnelian, and Chalcedony Tears. With the stone facing down, the grid opens the way for conception. Turned the other way, the Menalite holds a space for the project to gestate until it's time for its birth.

YOU WILL NEED:

- Template
- Keystone
- Six cleansing crystal points
- Six manifestation or conception crystals
- Six activation crystals
- Six anchor stones

TO LAY THE GRID:

1. Hold your crystals in your hands and state your intention for the grid.
2. Lay the keystone, restating your intention.
3. Lay the six cleansing crystal points on the narrow inner "petals" of the flower, pointing toward the center.
4. Lay the six manifestation or conception crystals at the outer ends of the inner "petals."
5. Lay the six activation crystals on the points of the larger "petals."
6. Use the power of your mind to connect the crystals and to light up the grid. Repeat your intention.
7. Lay the anchoring crystals on the outer perimeter, in line with the cleansing crystals on the inner petals.
8. Leave the grid in place and focus on it daily, keeping your project in mind. Remember to spray-cleanse it if the energy seems to be dissipating. Turn the grid if appropriate after conception occurs.
9. Remove the grid when the project comes to fruition or replace as appropriate.
10. After you have dismantled the grid by removing the crystals in the reverse order in which they were placed, cleanse them.

Grid-kit suggestions: Carnelian, Citrine, Chalcedony Tears, Fire Agate, Goldstone, Jade, Orange Kyanite, Menalite, Imperial Topaz, Shiva Lingam, Red Jasper. Cleansing crystals, anchoring crystals

ATTRACTING LOVE

We can never have too much love in our lives. This grid either attracts love and romance to you or strengthens a love relationship that already exists. It can be used to radiate love into the world, too. The heart grid is also the perfect forgiveness grid. You might use it to heal an old rift—say, between you and your partner or a friend—or even to send forgiveness to someone who's hurt you in the past.

This layout is a great example of how you can create your own grid. I was inspired to make it when I found a heart-shaped mount in an old photo frame in a junkshop.

Using the grid: Lay the grid to find new love, to strengthen old love, or to send unconditional love to the environment or a specific person.

Timing: The new moon is the traditional time to call in new love, but the grid can be laid at any time to radiate, restore, or strengthen affection.

Color and background: Pink, red, or green background. (Pink and red are associated with love and the heart, and green is associated with the heart chakra.)

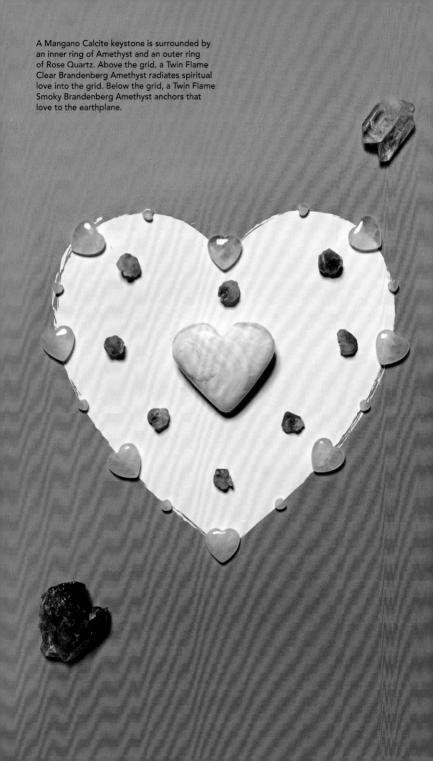

A Mangano Calcite keystone is surrounded by an inner ring of Amethyst and an outer ring of Rose Quartz. Above the grid, a Twin Flame Clear Brandenberg Amethyst radiates spiritual love into the grid. Below the grid, a Twin Flame Smoky Brandenberg Amethyst anchors that love to the earthplane.

YOU WILL NEED:

- Sufficient stones to outline the heart shape
- Keystone
- Anchor stone
- High-vibration Twin Flame stone (Twin Flame crystals are two crystals of roughly equal size joined together.)

TO LAY THE GRID:

1. Hold your crystals in your hands and state your intention for the grid.
2. Place crystals around the heart template, breathing mindfully as you do so.
3. If it feels appropriate, place an inner ring of heart stones.
4. Place an anchor stone at the base or wherever it feels most appropriate.
5. Place the keystone at the center or wherever it feels most appropriate.
6. Place a high-vibration Twin Flame stone above the grid.
7. Outline the heart with a crystal wand or join it with the power of your heart and mind.
8. Leave the grid in place for as long as it feels necessary to you to attract more love into your life. Remember to cleanse it regularly. Trust your intuition to tell you when to dismantle it.
9. When you're ready to dismantle your grid, remove the crystals in the reverse order in which they were laid, and cleanse them.

Grid-kit suggestions: Rose Quartz, Rhodochrosite, Rhodonite, Green Aventurine, Larimar, Selenite, Sugilite, Amazonite, Spirit Quartz, Soulmate formation (two crystals attached side by side). Anchor crystals. And see *Crystal Love/Love Crystals* in the Resources.

ABUNDANCE

A spiral draws energy into a stagnant situation or clears away negative energy. So, if your finances are floundering and you need an infusion of cash, use a spiral grid to clear away anything blocking your abundance—or, if you're seeking a raise or a new job, lay an abundance spiral. Place it over a lottery ticket or a scrap of paper with your wish printed on it. Abundance doesn't just involve money. Abundance is about feeling satisfied and secure with what you have, living an enriching and fulfilling life, sharing life's bounty, showing gratitude, and trusting that the universe will provide appropriately for all your needs.

Using the grid: First, lay the grid with the crystal points pointing up and out to cleanse the energies and remove any blockages to abundance. Cleanse your crystals, then switch, laying the grid with the crystals pointing in toward the center to draw in abundance.

Timing: New moon is the traditional time to begin new projects, but it is also customary to lay an abundance grid under a full moon. If time allows, lay a preparatory clearing grid first, as above, and then lay the second grid. (Remember to cleanse the crystals and the grid space in between.) Leave the grid in place for a moon cycle or until it has completed its work.

Color and background: Green, gold, and yellow are the traditional colors of abundance.

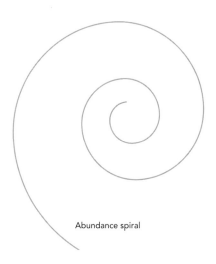

Abundance spiral

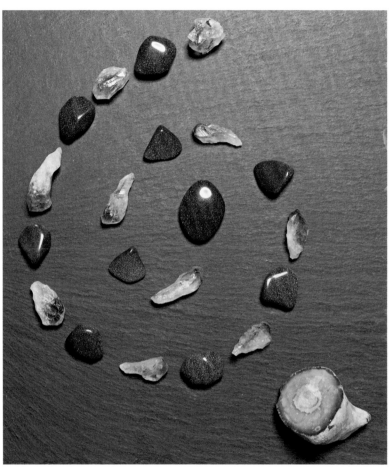

Abundance crystals are best placed on a base of petrified wood to ground them, but they can be laid as a spiral in the home, preferably on a wooden surface or rock base. This grid is laid on a slate base and utilizes a Flint anchor stone.

YOU WILL NEED:

- Base for the grid, such as wood, slate, fossilized wood, golden card, or golden cloth
- Cleansed and empowered Citrine and/or Goldstone
- Cleansed and empowered Herkimer Diamonds or Smoky Quartz
- Cleansed and empowered Goldstone for the keystone
- Anchor stone if appropriate

TO LAY THE GRID:

1. If you're laying a preparatory "cleansing" spiral, start at the topmost point and lay crystals alternately with the points pointing out from the center. Place the Goldstone in the center as the keystone. If laying an abundance grid, begin by placing the Goldstone in the center, stating that your intention is for it to bring abundance into your life.

2. Lay a spiral of alternated crystals, pointing down and inward, until you reach the Goldstone.

3. Add a grounding stone if appropriate.

4. When the grid is no longer required, dismantle it.

Grid-kit suggestions: Citrine, Goldstone, Green Aventurine, Herkimer Diamond, Jade, Moss Agate, Ruby, Tiger's Eye, Topaz

CAREER AND LIFEPATH

Although Metatron's Cube looks complex at first glance, it only takes two sets of carefully positioned crystals and a central keystone to clarify complicated situations and take you to the heart of what really matters. Be aware, though, that the answers may present themselves in an unusual, unexpected fashion. Metatron's Cube can also be used to help you to gain promotion and advance in your chosen field.

Using the grid: If you are unsure of which path to follow in life, particularly in relation to your career, lay the grid and ask for guidance. Affirm that the perfect opportunity manifests with perfect timing. If you are seeking promotion, lay the grid before approaching your boss with the request or before interviewing for a new position.

Timing: Ideally, you should lay the Cube at a new moon and expect an answer by the full moon. Afterward, the grid can be dismantled.

Color and background: Gold, silver, or a color that is compatible with your intended career. For example, if you were in medicine, you might choose blue, the traditional color of healing; or, if you were in banking, you might choose yellow or gold to represent abundance or money. A natural base of stone or wood is practical and pragmatic, too, grounding the answer in the everyday.

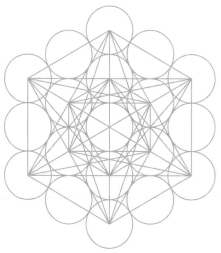

Metatron's Cube

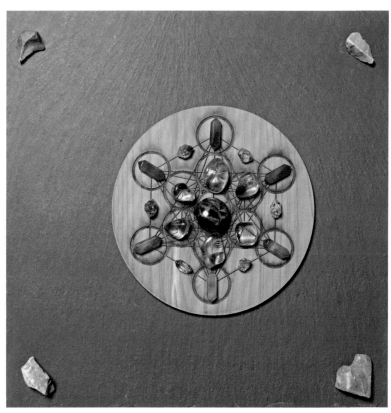

A tumbled Pietersite for insight is surrounded by tumbled Citrine, Smoky Herkimer Diamonds, and Carnelian points. The grid is anchored with Flint.

YOU WILL NEED:

- Template
- Six career and/or lifepath crystals
- Six grounding crystals
- Keystone
- Crystal wand

TO LAY THE GRID:

1. Hold your crystals in your hands and state your intention for the grid.
2. Lay six career or lifepath crystals around the central hexagon.
3. Lay six grounding stones around the outer hexagon.
4. Add additional clearing stones around the perimeter if appropriate.
5. Lay the keystone in the center to fire up the grid.
6. Move a crystal wand from each of the outer crystals into the center. (Use a crystal wand for this grid, as it is complex and best joined with a wand to clarify the energy flow.) Restate your intention.
7. Breathe steadily for a few moments, focusing your eyes on the grid. Then gently disconnect from it, and leave it undisturbed in your environment, letting it do its work. Leave the grid in place until you receive your answer.
8. When you're ready to dismantle your grid, remove the crystals in the reverse order in which they were laid, then cleanse them.

Grid-kit suggestions: Blue Jade, Carnelian, Citrine, Green Aventurine, Green Tourmaline, Moss Agate, Rose Quartz, Turquoise, Tiger's Eye, Septarian. Grounding crystals.
Lifepath crystals: Eudialyte, Turquoise, Strawberry Lemurian Seed, Pietersite, "Life Path" crystal (which is long, thin, and clear, with one or more absolutely smooth sides)

TRANQUILITY

The Flower of Life is essentially a grid of tranquility. It radiates peace and goodwill into the environment, and you can lay on it any intuitive pattern that feels right to you. It is best laid on the template so that the underlying geometry connects the crystals. That way, you don't need to place one on every single point. Lay the Flower of Life if you think you may be coming to the end of a tumultuous period in your life and want to invite calm and tranquility into your daily experience or if you're surrounded by upheaval and stress in your home or workplace—due, perhaps, to rebellious teenage children or to pressure from your boss.

Using the grid: Choose a place where the grid will not be disturbed and leave it to do its work.

Timing: No specific timing.

Color and background: The Flower of Life can be laid on any color or background material but using wood or other natural materials helps the peaceful energy to anchor itself. Beautiful, purpose-made boards are readily available.

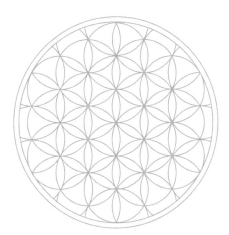

Flower of Life

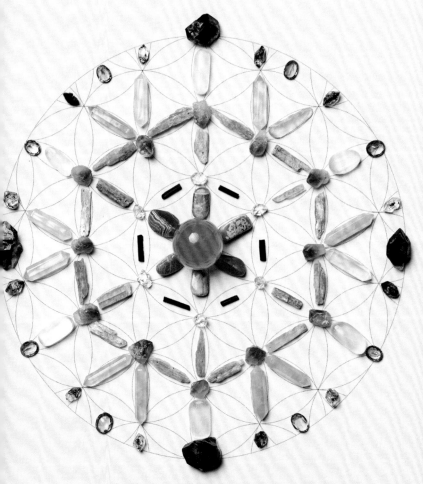

This sphere of tranquility centers around Rose Quartz and Rhodochrosite, outlined by Black Tourmaline and Herkimer Diamonds. The
green circle is Kyanite interspersed with Amethyst, surrounded further
by Rose Quartz and Selenite. The outer circle is Amethyst, and Smoky
Quartz anchor the cardinal points.

YOU WILL NEED:

- Template
- Sufficient crystals to lay the pattern you choose on the grid (Dowse or use your intuition to select your crystals.)
- At least one anchor stone (ideally four to six)
- Keystone

TO LAY THE GRID:

1. Hold the crystals in your hands and state your intention for the grid.
2. Begin by laying the keystone in the center and restating your intention.
3. Create a pattern around the Flower of Life, placing at least one anchor stone on the outer ring, but preferably four to six. (You can create any pattern you like within the grid. For example, you could create only a single central flower, if that feels right to you, or you could fill in the whole outer ring of petals.)
4. Place light-bringing crystals around the perimeter.
5. Leave the grid in place to do its work for as long as necessary—permanently, if required.
6. To dismantle this grid, simply remove the crystals—the energy will dissipate on its own after the crystals are removed, so no cleansing is needed.

Grid-kit suggestions: Rose Quartz, Selenite, Rhodochrosite, Quartz, Labradorite, Kyanite, Eye of the Storm (Judy's Jasper), Smoky Quartz

JOY AND REJUVENATION

Lay the Joy and Rejuvenation grid to revitalize your daily experience or to bring about social change and regeneration. This joyful grid demonstrates just how color can affect and interact with a grid. Use bright pink stones instead of the green in the Tranquility Grid. The Flower of Life radiates joy and rejuvenation into an area that has become energetically dead. That may be into a part of your own life or that of a community, into over-cultivated soil, or even into a whole country. It is helpful for a community that has grown apathetic following a loss, shock, or trauma and which needs to regenerate itself. The grid enthusiastically activates the energies and gets things moving. It is particularly helpful where depression and hopelessness have taken over, or if you're surrounded by apathy in the workplace or in community matters, as it also strengthens motivation and a desire to get things done. You don't have to be personally involved to lend energetic support in this way. Color-coated crystals were chosen to infuse vitality, as this vibrant color is difficult to source as points in a natural form. This joyful grid is best laid on a template so that the underlying geometry connects the crystals and radiates the energies outward.

Form: On the Flower of Life background, lay any shape that intuitively feels right to you.

Using the grid: Choose a place where the grid will not be disturbed and leave it to do its work.

Timing: No specific timing.

Color and background: Anchoring and radiating material such as wood, slate, or the earth helps the rejuvenating energy to ground itself in the everyday world. Bright-colored backgrounds assist in spreading the joy. Beautiful, purpose-made boards are readily available.

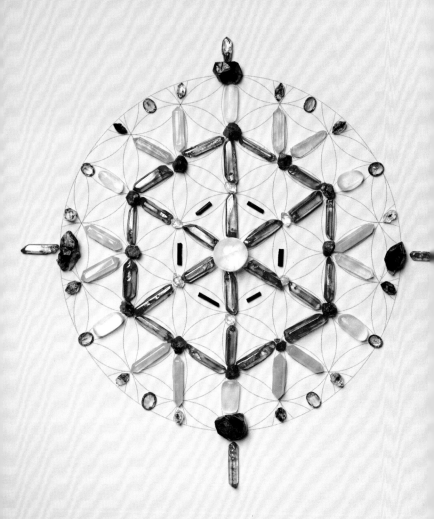

This joy and rejuvenation grid centers around a Selenite ball and coated Rose Aura
Quartz outlined by Black Tourmaline and Herkimer Diamonds. Rose Aura "petals"
lead to a Rose Aura circle interspersed with natural Rhodolite Garnets. The next
petal circle combines Rose Quartz and Selenite. The outer circle is Amethyst, Smoky
Herkimers, and double terminated Smoky Quartz to anchor the cardinal points, with
further Rose Aura points to direct the energy out into the community.

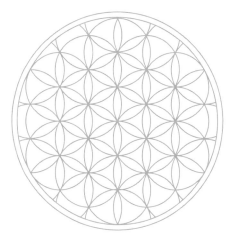

Flower of Life

YOU WILL NEED:

- Template
- Sufficient crystals to lay the pattern (Dowse to select your crystals or use your intuition.)
- At least one anchor stone (ideally four to six)
- Keystone

TO LAY THE GRID:

1. Hold the crystals in your hands and state your intention for the grid.
2. Begin by laying the keystone in the center and restating your intention.
3. Create a pattern around the keystone, placing at least one anchor stone on the outer ring, but preferably four to six.
4. Place appropriate crystals around the perimeter.
5. Leave the grid in place to do its work for as long as necessary—permanently, if required.
6. To dismantle this grid, simply remove the crystals—the energy will slowly dissipate on its own after the crystals are removed, so no cleansing is required.

Grid-kit suggestions: Rose or Ruby Aura Quartz, Cobalto Calcite, Rhodolite Garnet, Erythrite, Rose Quartz, Selenite, Quartz, Herkimer Diamond, Red Kyanite, Poppy Jasper, Hematite Quartz *Anchoring:* Eye of the Storm (Judy's Jasper), Polychrome Jasper, Smoky Quartz, Hematite, Red Flint

CHILDREN

The Fruit of Life, which is contained within the Flower of Life, helps to support children and bring out their highest potential by creating a stable environment for them. This grid can be tailored to an individual child's needs. The central ring of crystals can be changed to help them meet the challenges they face, so this grid can be left in place long term. Children enjoy being with crystals, so actively involve them in choosing and laying the grid crystals—always under your supervision, of course—and place grids out of the reach of small children.

Using the grid: The grid can be laid in an older child's or teenager's room, but a grid for young children should always be placed high up out of reach.

Timing: The grid can be laid at any time, but it is particularly useful when a child is facing any kind of challenge or exhibiting challenging behavior.

Color and background: Choose a color that is supportive and calming for the child's challenge or issue. For instance, if your child struggles with reading and writing, lay a dyslexia grid on pale creamy yellow (research shows that brown text on cream paper is easier for a dyslexic child to read). If your child is being bullied, a soft pink base softens the aggression, while a pale orange one supports the courage the child needs to overcome this.

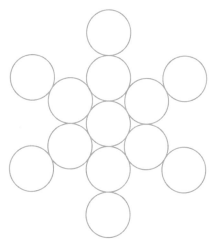

Fruit of Life

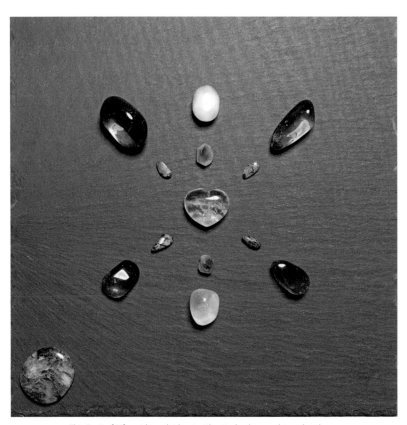

This Fruit of Life grid was laid out without a background template by a child who was struggling to learn to read. The anchor stone is Sugilite, which also surrounds the central Quartz heart that the child chose to represent himself together with Amethyst for mental clarity. Smoky Quartz and Selenite acted as anchors and light-bringers.

YOU WILL NEED:

- Central keystone to represent your child
- Six "issue" or calming stones
- Four grounding crystals
- Two light-bringing crystals

TO LAY THE GRID:

1. Hold your crystals in your hands and state your intention for the grid.
2. Lay the central keystone to represent your child.
3. Lay six crystals around the keystone to assist with the challenge or issue.
   (These crystals can either represent a single issue, or different ones—whichever feels best to you. However, it may be more effective to address separate issues by laying individual grids.)
4. Lay four grounding crystals to anchor the grid at each corner of the "square."
5. Lay a light-bringing crystal at the top and bottom.
6. Leave in place until the issue or issues have been resolved, remembering to cleanse the grid regularly.

Grid-kit suggestions: Crackle Quartz, Pink Agate, Coprolite ("Dinosaur Poo"), Fuchsite, Howlite, Rose Quartz, Turquenite, Youngite *Examinations and concentration:* Orange Kyanite, Fluorite, Rose Quartz, Green Aventurine *Communication:* Blue Lace Agate, Pink Agate, Blue Crackle Quartz, Youngite, Chinese Writing Stone, Chrysanthemum Stone, Sodalite

Autism: Muscovite, Sugilite, Charoite, Moldavite, Fuchsite, Sodalite, Lapis Lazuli, Amethyst, Lepidolite, Turquoise *ADHD:* Lepidolite, Lithium Quartz, Kunzite, Rutilated Quartz *Dyslexia:* Sugilite, Blue Crackle Quartz, Sodalite, Fuchsite, Emerald Quartz, Amethyst *Dyspraxia:* Black Moonstone, Sugilite, Lepidolite, Muscovite, Cherry Quartz *Temper tantrums:* Rose Quartz, Blue Lace Agate, Howlite, Pink Crackle Quartz, Rose Aura Quartz *Nightmares:* Chrysoprase, Amethyst, Prehnite, Bloodstone.

HARMONIOUS RELATIONSHIPS

The Vesica Piscis brings people together in harmonious relationships—and that's not limited only to marriages or other romantic partnerships. This grid is also advantageous for work colleagues, friends, business associates, and anyone else in your life with whom you've had a misunderstanding or need to harmonize ideas.

Using the grid: Lay the grid whenever you want to bring two people together for mutual benefit or to soothe disagreements.

Timing: No specific timing.

Color and background: A pink background works well for the Vesica Piscis. If a relationship needs grounding in the everyday rather than the fantasy world, lay it on a natural material, such as stone or wood.

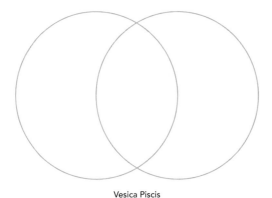

Vesica Piscis

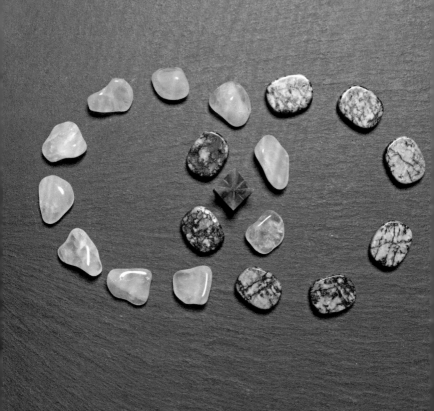

YOU WILL NEED:

- Sufficient crystals to outline the two circles
- Shiva Lingam or another appropriate keystone

TO LAY THE GRID:

1. Hold your crystals in your hands and state your intention for the grid.
2. Outline the left-hand circle in crystals first.
3. Outline the right-hand (overlapping) circle next.
4. Place the keystone in the center and restate your intention.
5. Leave in place for as long as you feel is necessary to keep the relationship on track, cleansing the grid regularly.
6. To dismantle the grid, remove the crystals in the order in which they were laid, then cleanse them.

Grid-kit suggestions: Rose Quartz, Selenite, Smoky Quartz, Rhodochrosite, Rhodonite, Green Aventurine, Agate, Watermelon Tourmaline, Pink and Green Tourmalines, Turquoise, Shiva Lingam, Twin Flame (two crystals springing side by side from the same base)

Rose Quartz and Rhodonite circles around a Green Aventurine Merkaba keystone restore unconditional love to a mature partnership.

PERSON TO PERSON

Grids can be used to send distant healing or support to a specific person. The grid is laid over the name or a photograph of the person. A combination of healing and clearing crystals ensures that the healing energies gently balance the person's energy field.

Using the grid: This grid should only be used with the permission of the person concerned. If he or she is too ill or is out of contact, ask that healing be available to him or her for their highest good and benefit—but only if this is appropriate. (If in doubt, dowse to find out whether it is appropriate.)

Timing: No specific timing.

Color and background: Blue is the traditional color of healing.

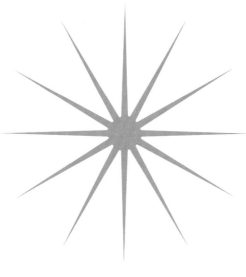

Sunburst

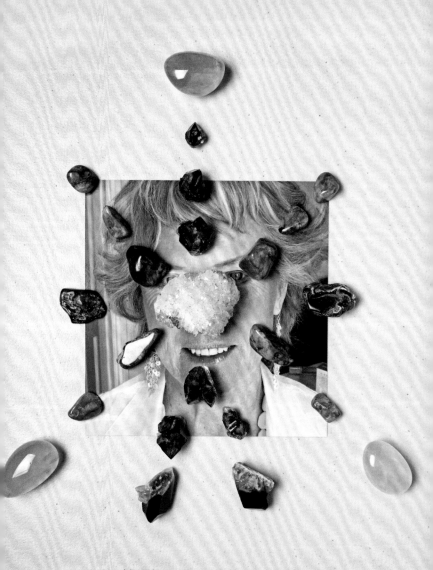

An Anandalite™ keystone surrounded by a sunburst of Smoky Quartz, Quantum Quattro, Eye of the Storm (Judy's Jasper), and Rose Quartz sent continual healing and support to a dear friend.

YOU WILL NEED:

- Sufficient healing and clearing crystals to create the sunburst
- Keystone appropriate to the condition or need

TO LAY THE GRID:

1. Hold the crystals in your hands and state your intention for the grid: namely, that appropriate healing will flow to the person named [insert name] *in the best way possible.*
2. Lay a keystone in the center of the photograph or over the person's name.
3. Lay alternate rows of clearing crystals (pointing outward, if the crystals have points) and rows of healing crystals (pointing inward if the crystals have points).
4. Use the power of your mind to activate the grid. Watch it fire up, clearing and unblocking stuck energies and bringing the person back into balance. (Do not join up the grid—the energy needs to radiate to the person in question.) If the person is ungrounded, you can lay a perimeter of grounding stones, if appropriate. (Dowse or use your intuition to find out whether this is the case.)
5. Leave the grid in place for as long as necessary, or until the issue is resolved. When you're ready, dismantle the grid.

Grid-kit suggestions: *Clearing crystals:* Smoky Quartz, Black Tourmaline, Shungite *Healing crystals:* Quantum Quattro, Bloodstone, Que Sera, Amethyst, Quartz, Klinoptilolith, Scolecite with Natrolite.

ANCESTRAL

The Celtic Tree of Life is the perfect layout for healing the ancestral line and sending healing forward into future generations. It breaks old patterns, switches off detrimental energetic potential in the subtle DNA, and switches on beneficial energetic potential in the DNA, taking the crystal energy deep within the family and between the cells of the physical body.

Using the grid: Use this layout if there has been family and intergenerational trauma or toxic emotions or ingrained patterns carried down through the ancestral line. You can lay it on and around your own body to act as a surrogate for the ancestors and future generations.

Timing: This grid is particularly effective when laid at the dark of the moon and left in place until a full moon. It can also be laid at the winter solstice and can remain in place until the summer solstice, provided it is regularly cleansed and tended as appropriate.

Color and background: A green cloth and/or natural materials, such as wood or stone.

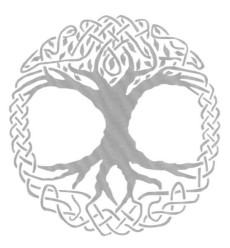

Celtic Tree of Life

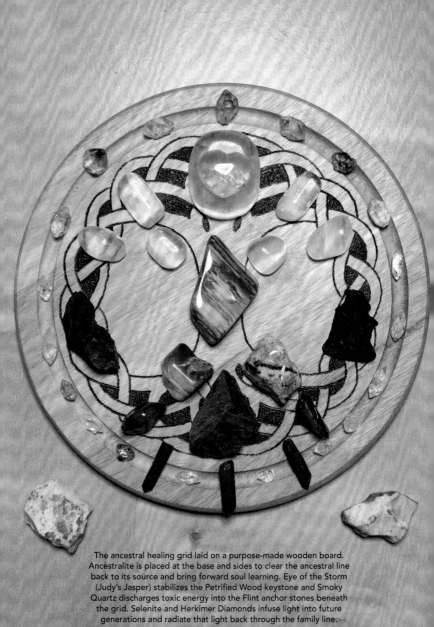

The ancestral healing grid laid on a purpose-made wooden board. Ancestralite is placed at the base and sides to clear the ancestral line back to its source and bring forward soul learning. Eye of the Storm (Judy's Jasper) stabilizes the Petrified Wood keystone and Smoky Quartz discharges toxic energy into the Flint anchor stones beneath the grid. Selenite and Herkimer Diamonds infuse light into future generations and radiate that light back through the family line.

YOU WILL NEED:

- Sufficient crystals for the trunk and base to represent the present-life family
- Sufficient ancestral or grounding and detoxifying crystals for the roots, to represent the ancestors
- Sufficient light-bringing crystals for the branches to represent future generations
- Keystone

TO LAY THE GRID:

1. Hold your crystals in your hands and state your intention for the grid.
2. Place appropriate crystals on the trunk to represent the present-life family.
3. Place the ancestral or grounding and detoxifying crystals or anchor stones on the roots.
4. Place the light-bringing crystals in the branches to represent future generations.
5. Place an anchor stone in the base of the trunk and a keystone above.
6. Use the power of your mind to activate the grid—without connecting it up—and to send healing into the past and to future generations.
7. To dismantle the grid, remove the stones in the reverse order in which they were placed. (There's no need to use sound or clearing essence for dismantling this particular grid. You can leave its energy to continue working, even after it's been dismantled.)

Grid-kit suggestions: Ancestralite, Brandenberg Amethyst, Cradle of Life (Humankind), Freedom Stone, Kambaba Jasper, Celtic Quartz, Petrified Wood, Preseli Bluestone, Stromatolite, Chrysotile, Dumortierite, Selenite, Petalite, crystals from the ancestral homeland

SITUATIONAL

The triple spiral layout can be used in a similar fashion to a three-card Tarot spread. It highlights and heals not only the present situation, but also its origins. In this grid, the bottom right-hand spiral represents the present situation; the left-hand spiral reveals and heals the underlying causes behind the situation; and the top spiral ensures a beneficial outcome. It can be used for healing family rifts, for work situations, for friendships, or for the benefit of the wider world.

Using the grid: Use this grid to assist any situation that requires healing and resolution.

Timing: This grid can be laid at any time, but it is particularly potent to lay the right-hand spiral at the dark of the moon; the left-hand one at a new moon; and the top spiral at a full moon. Leave in place until the following dark moon or until the situation has resolved itself.

Color and background: Choose an appropriate color and background for the type of situation involved. Use your intuition, or dowse to decide on color and background.

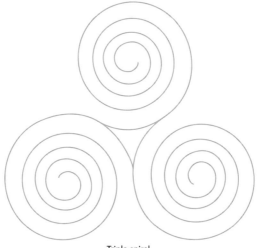

Triple spiral

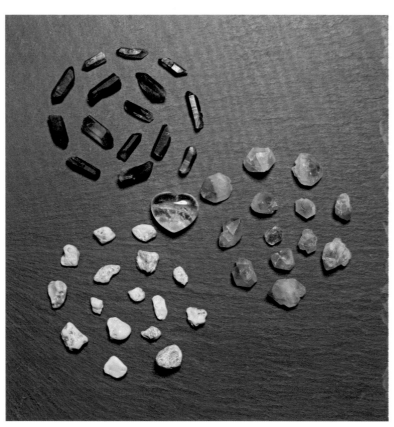

Spirals of Smoky Quartz, Turquoise, and Amethyst surround a Quartz heart to heal a lack of communication caused by misunderstanding of the core issues and a clash of opposing viewpoints.

YOU WILL NEED:

- Template
- Sufficient crystals for each spiral
- Keystone

TO LAY THE GRID:

1. Hold the crystals for the first spiral in your hands and state your intention for the grid.
2. Lay the right-hand spiral from the center outward. Pointed crystals should be placed point-outward from the center.
3. Use the power of your mind to join up the crystals, moving from the center of the spiral to the center point of the triple spiral.
4. Lay the keystone in the center, restating your intention.
5. Cleanse the grid (but leave it in place, so that you can add spirals during the course of the development of the grid). Lay the second and third spirals in turn as appropriate, connecting to the central keystone each time.
6. Leave the grid in place until the time comes to dismantle it, remembering to cleanse it regularly.

Grid-kit suggestions: *Conflict resolution:* Spirit Quartz, Elestial Quartz, Chalcedony, Chrysocolla, Green Agate, Jade, Picture Jasper, Prehnite, Rose Quartz, Shiva Lingam, Rutilated or Tourminalated Quartz, Strawberry Quartz, Indicolite Quartz, Watermelon Tourmaline *Cleansing:* Shungite, Smoky Quartz, Black Tourmaline, Hematite *Light-bringing:* Anandalite™, Petalite, Phenacite, Selenite

ON A MAP

The hexagram layout is extremely stabilizing, so it is particularly appropriate when there has been an upheaval of the earth in a local environment, such as an earthquake or a tsunami. Placed over a map, it facilitates rebalancing and healing the land. Since it is a clearing and transmuting grid, it can also assist in areas where there has been ancestral trauma—such as sites of concentration camps or other areas where ethnic cleansing has taken place—or land clearing, as in the Amazon rainforests.

Using the grid: Lay the grid where it will not be disturbed. Leave it in place until the situation resolves.

Timing: Use this grid whenever there has been upheaval in the local environment or to assist such a situation anywhere in the world—in which case, place the crystals on a map.

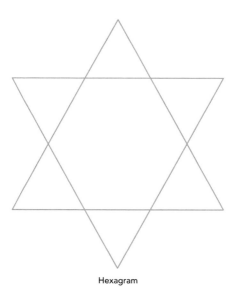

Hexagram

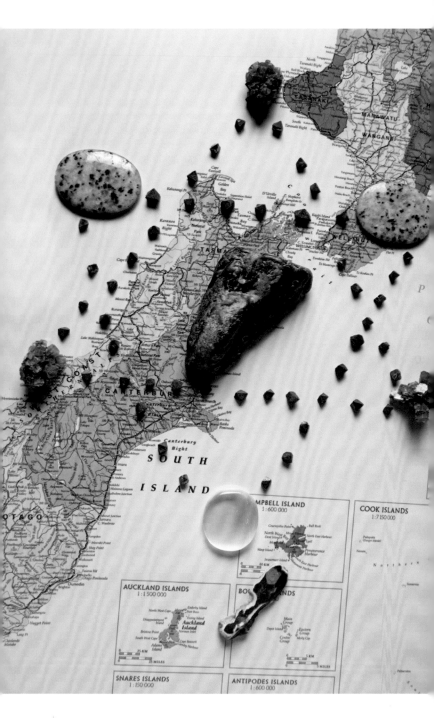

YOU WILL NEED:

- Three clearing crystals
- Three earth-healing or light-bringing crystals
- Keystone
- Anchor stones
- Additional crystals as appropriate

TO LAY THE GRID:

1. Hold your crystals in your hands and state your intention for the grid.
2. Lay the upward-pointing triangle with clearing crystals first.
3. Then lay the downward-pointing triangle with healing or light-bringing crystals.
4. Place the keystone in the center and restate your intention.
5. Anchor the grid if appropriate. Dowse or use your intuition to find out whether this is so and which crystals to use.
6. Cleanse the grid regularly and substitute or place additional crystals if appropriate. Leave in place until the situation has been resolved.
7. To dismantle the grid, remove the stones in the reverse order in which they were placed. (There's no need to use sound or clearing essence for dismantling this particular grid. You can happily leave its energy to continue working, even after it's been dismantled.)

Grid-kit suggestions: Anandalite™, Aragonite, Jade, Kiwi Jasper, Magnetite, Smoky Quartz, Rhodozite, Rose Quartz, Quartz, Selenite, Ruby in Kyanite or Zoisite, Smoky Quartz, Hematite, local stones

Following the recurrence of severe earthquakes in the Christchurch area of New Zealand in 2016, a keystone of Pounamou Jade from the local Greenstone trail was laid over the site on a map. An anchoring grid of Rhodozite was laid around it. Kiwi Jasper and Selenite brought in comfort and light to the traumatized inhabitants, and Aragonite sputniks stabilized the equally traumatized land.

CRYSTAL GLOSSARY

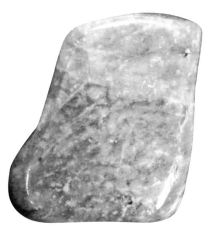

AMAZONITE

Amazonite shields the body from the effects of subtle radiation and electromagnetic frequencies, including WiFi, which depletes the immune systems in sensitive people. The stone also aligns the subtle nervous system with the physical nervous system and relieves muscle spasms.

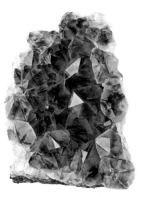

AMETHYST

Amethyst opens your third eye and clarifies spiritual vision. By creating a safe sacred space for meditation and multi-dimensional exploration, it clears your mind and aids enlightenment. By detaching you from unwanted entities, thought forms, or mental constructs, Amethyst dispels illusions that prevent you from experiencing true reality. It helps you dream a new world into being.

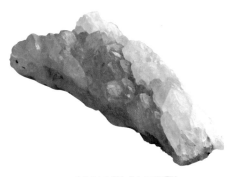

ANANDALITE™

An exceedingly high vibration crystal, Anandalite™ draws down cosmic wisdom and connects to celestial beings and the archangels.

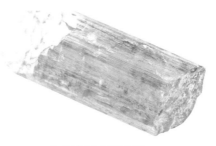

AQUAMARINE

Aquamarine assists in letting go of mental constructs and underlying emotional states. It reminds you that progress is the law of life—the soul must evolve along the pathway it laid down for itself prior to incarnation.

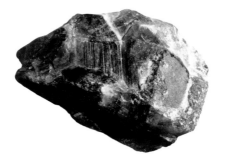

AURALITE 23

This extremely high vibration, multi-layered crystal brings profound peace and clarity, containing the wisdom of the ages.

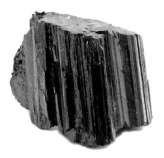

BLACK TOURMALINE

Most Black Tourmaline contains iron, making it
a powerfully protective stone. Due to its inner structure,
however, Tourmaline traps negative energy within it
rather than bouncing it back and forth as iron-based
stones are prone to do. Use it in a grid around your
home to create a protective shield that blocks negativity
or toxic energy of any kind.

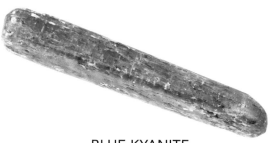

BLUE KYANITE

Tranquil Blue Kyanite is one of the few crystals that
do not hold onto negative energy (but it should
nevertheless be cleansed). Its high vibrations rapidly
transfer energy and create new energetic and neural
pathways, acting like a universal bridge. It opens
metaphysical abilities and activates the higher chakras,
aligning them with the subtle bodies.

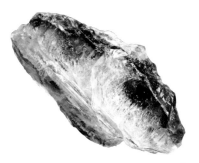

BRANDENBERG AMETHYST

The Brandenberg Amethyst brings about deep soul
healing and forgiveness. It is the finest tool available
for removing implants, attachments, spirit possession,
or mental influence; this is the stone excellent for
transformation or transition.

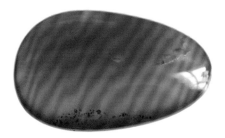

CARNELIAN

Carnelian stimulates courage and action. It restores
motivation, energizes the soul body, and helps turn
dreams into realities. With this stone, you can work an
act of truly outrageous magic that transmogrifies the
mundane world. For instance, use it to successfully apply
for a dream job for which you are not qualified.

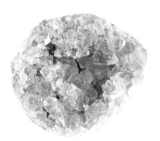

CELESTITE

One of the major angel connectors, Celestite stimulates
clairvoyance and promotes dream recall and out-of-body
journeys. It teaches you how to trust the infinite wisdom
of the universe. A crystal for conflict resolution, it instills
balance in times of stress.

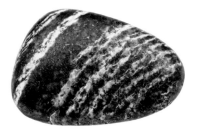

CHRYSOTILE

Chrysotile links you to the knowledge of the ages. This
stone helps you clear away the debris of the past to reveal
your core Self. It also works on the etheric blueprint to
correct imbalances and blockages that could manifest as
disease. Toxic—always use tumbled.

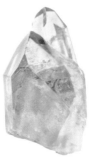

CITRINE

Citrine gives you energy to manifest your own reality and to attract everything you need. It invigorates the body and activates the immune system. Beneficial for degenerative dis-eases, it encourages energy flow and balances hormones.

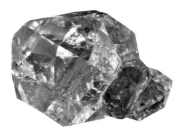

CLEAR HERKIMER DIAMOND

Herkimers transform the way you see the world. They aid you in creating new neural pathways within the physical body that connect to the lightbody and to All That Is to manifest your spiritual potential on earth. Herkimer attunes you to a much higher reality and accelerates your spiritual growth, so you become coherent at every level of being.

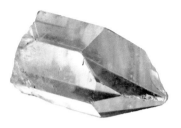

CLEAR QUARTZ

Clear Quartz works on multi-dimensional
levels of being. Generating electromagnetism and
dispelling static electricity, it is an extremely powerful
healing and energy amplifier.

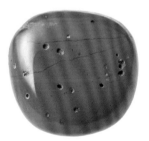

CORAL

Coral is not a crystal, but it is highly charged with
passionate Qi, especially in its red form. It has been
a living organism and should be used judiciously. It
traditionally assists blood and circulatory system issues
and enhances vitality. *Note:* As Coral is an endangered
species, ensure that you buy ethically sourced Coral that
has not been obtained from a living reef.

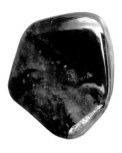

CRADLE OF LIFE (HUMANKIND)

Rock from the cave where the first human ancestral bones
were discovered, Cradle of Life takes you back to first
principles and root causes. It rebuilds your sense of self,
inputting newer, more appropriate patterns.

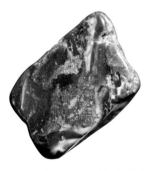

EYE OF THE STORM
(JUDY'S JASPER)

Eye of the Storm gives you core stability in which to
calmly ride out changes and challenges. It reminds you
that the bigger picture is ever changing, offering an
objective perspective on how your actions could affect
the outcome. This stone instills a deep sense of self-worth
from which to interact with the outside world.

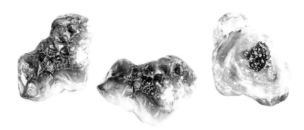

FIRE AGATE

Fire Agate facilitates the evolution of consciousness.
It clears etheric blockages and energizes the aura. Fire
Agate has a deep connection to the earth and its energy is
calming, bringing security and safety.

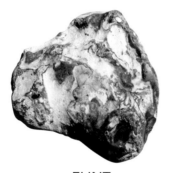

FLINT

Flint assists detoxification and pain release. Its power heals at
emotional, psychological, and energetic levels rather than physical.
Metaphorically, it cuts through blockages, past-life ties, and chakra
connections that you have outgrown. Taking you deep into yourself,
Flint reveals and transmutes underlying causes of depression. It assists
you in bringing your shadow's gifts into conscious awareness. It creates
core stability and restructures information stored in the cells. By cutting
away all that no longer serves you, it sets you free from the past.

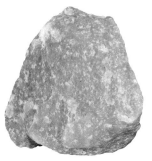

GREEN AVENTURINE

Green Aventurine protects the spleen chakra from energy vampires and protects against EMF emissions. It is a great stone to accompany you outside your comfort zone, as it provides courage and encouragement.

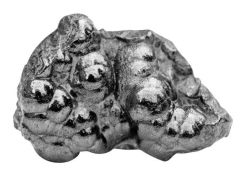

HEMATITE

Useful for past-life healings that involve war, wounds, and bloodshed, this powerful stone also assists in overcoming addictions rooted in emotional cravings or unfulfilled desires. Hold Hematite to ground the soul back into your body after journeying or after spiritual work.

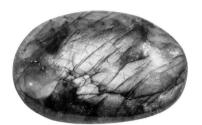

LABRADORITE

Labradorite provides a protective shield between
you and the outside world. Stimulating metaphysical
gifts, it reaches into multidimensions to contact
the spiritual world.

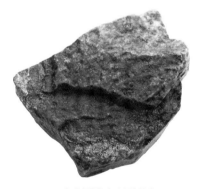

LAPIS LAZULI

Lapis Lazuli is a key to spiritual attainment. Enhancing
dreamwork and metaphysical abilities, it facilitates
spiritual journeying and stimulates personal and spiritual
power. By transmuting mental and emotional blockages,
Lapis sets your soul free to express itself fully.

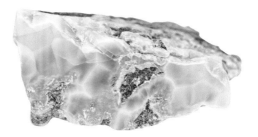

LARIMAR

Serene Blue Larimar provides freedom from self-imposed
limitations and creates a sense of peace through finding
truth. It can be used for multi-dimensional and cellular
work and tfor stimulating the heart and higher chakras.

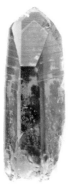

LEMURIAN SEED

An extremely effective connector and activator for grids,
Lemurian Seed crystal has an exceptionally high vibration
that assists in the evolution of the planet. It contains
knowledge from ancient Lemuria and beyond.

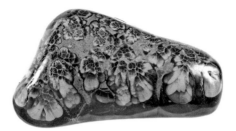

MALACHITE

Malachite is a power stone for intense inner transformation and soul catharsis. This crystal is merciless in exposing personality imperfections, outgrown patterns, blockages, and ties that must be dissolved before you can evolve spiritually. It requires you to take responsibility for your thoughts, feelings, and actions. This makes it an excellent karmic and soul cleanser, activating your soul's purpose.

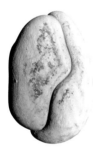

MENALITE

The perfect stone to accompany all the transitions of womanhood, Menalite is excellent for stimulating conception and assisting birth in all its forms. It maintains hormonal balance and removes fear of death.

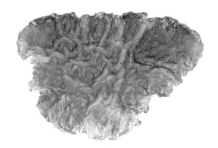

MOLDAVITE

A meteorite flew in from outer space and fused with the
ground on which it landed, uniting heaven and earth
to create Moldavite. This high-vibration crystal links
"above" and "below," accessing the Akashic record and
All That Is (source energy).

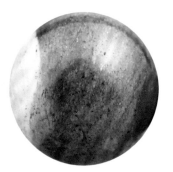

MOOKAITE JASPER

Mookaite is an excellent substitute for Coral.
This highly potent crystal infuses the body with
vitality and either sedates (yellow) or stimulates (red)
the immune system as required.

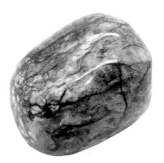

PIETERSITE

Pietersite promotes "walking your truth." It can be used for a vision quest or shamanic journey and it accesses a high state of altered awareness. It removes conditioning imposed by other people and links you to your inner guidance.

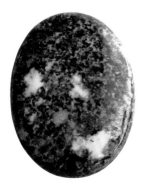

PRESELI BLUESTONE

Powerfully magnetic, Preseli Bluestone provides an inner compass to show you the way. It grounds healing energy into the planet or the body and is a powerful antidote to EMF emissions.

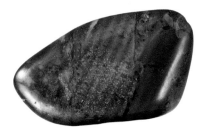

RED JASPER

Connected with the base chakra, courageous
Red Jasper is a physically invigorating stone that imparts
vitality and optimism. It replenishes lost energy and can
energize a whole grid.

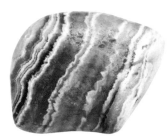

RHODOCHROSITE

One of the major healing "love stones," Rhodochrosite
encourages the expression of feelings and encourages
forgiveness of the past. This compassionate stone draws
love to you and comforts those who are alone.

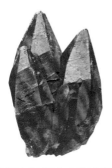

ROSE AURA QUARTZ

Rose Aura Quartz works to transmute deeply held doubts about self-worth, bestowing the gift of unconditional love of yourself and making a powerful connection to universal love.

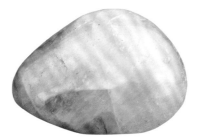

ROSE QUARTZ

Rose Quartz heals emotions and transforms relationships with yourself and others, drawing in love and harmony. This crystal of auric and heart protection brings loving vibes into your heart and into your subtle etheric bodies. At a metaphysical level, Rose Quartz stimulates the third eye, strengthening scrying power and opening clairvoyance to the finest levels of guidance.

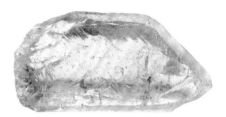

SELENITE

Selenite accesses angelic consciousness and brings divine light into everything it touches. A powerful transmutor for emotional energy, Selenite releases core feelings behind psychosomatic illnesses and emotional blockages.

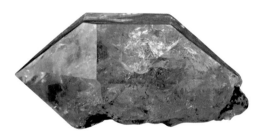

SMOKY HERKIMER DIAMOND

Smoky Herkimer is a high-vibration stone and an excellent psychic clearing tool. It protects against electromagnetic or geopathic pollution.

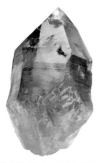

SMOKY QUARTZ

This versatile healing crystal carries the underlying properties of Quartz. It works on the kidneys and other organs of elimination to remove toxins from the body. An excellent grounding stone for rebalancing the body, Smoky Quartz strengthens underlying core stability and prevents healing crises from occurring. In a healing grid, Smoky Quartz absorbs disharmonious environmental energy. With the point facing out, it transmutes negative energy and draws in healing light.

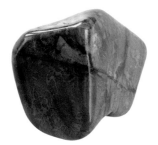

SUGILITE

A natural tranquilizer, gentle Sugilite is particularly helpful for children—or anyone—who feel like misfits. It prevents bullying and assists with reading capacity.

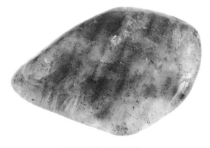

SUNSTONE

A powerfully energizing stone, Sunstone infuses the light
of the sun into an area or a physical body, revitalizing
it instantly. It is particularly useful in the dark days of
winter. Use it to attract abundance.

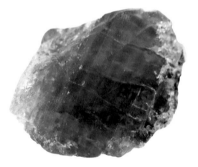

TANZANITE

High-vibration Tanzanite facilitates altered states of
consciousness and stimulates metaphysical abilities,
linking to archangels and Ascended Masters. Accelerating
spiritual growth, it downloads information from the
Akashic record to dissolve outdated karmic dis-ease.

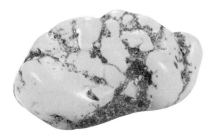

TURQUOISE

Turquoise lets you explore past lives to find the primary source of a martyred attitude or self-sabotage. If you are pessimistic, it teaches you to focus on solutions rather than problems or the past. This stone dispels negative belief patterns and removes toxic energy, reminding you that you are a spiritual being who happens to be having a human learning experience.

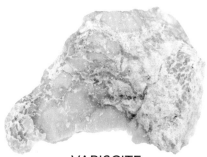

VARISCITE

Helpful for past life exploration, Variscite facilitates visual images while going deeply into the feelings of appropriate lives, stimulating insight and helping one reframe situations. This stone facilitates moving out of deep despair and into a position of trust with the Universe.

GLOSSARY

Arc: A section of the circumference of a circle or a curving trajectory. An arc can also be a sustained luminous discharge of electricity or energy across a gap in a circuit or between electrodes (or crystals).

Astrological elements and triplicities: The zodiac is divided into a series of four equilateral triangles, and each triangle contains the three signs in each element: fire, which represents spirit and creativity; air, which represents inspiration and ideas; earth, which represents pragmatic grounding; and water, which represents emotions and intuition. Within each elemental group, one sign is cardinal; one is fixed; and one is mutable. For example, within the triangle that contains the Earth signs, Taurus is fixed; Virgo is mutable; and Capricorn is cardinal. Cardinal, fixed, and mutable describe how easily and quickly energy and change flow through a sign. "Cardinal" is the initiating energy; "fixed" is the consolidating force; and "mutable" refers to the ability to adapt and go with the flow. So, the first triplicity in the zodiac is fire, in which Aries is cardinal, Leo is fixed, and Sagittarius is mutable.

Dis-ease: A state of energetic disharmony created by a discordant environment, toxic emotions, and ingrained thought patterns. Unless it is healed, dis-ease can lead to physical or mental disturbances.

Electromagnetic smog/EMFs: A subtle but detectable electromagnetic field produced by power lines and electrical equipment that has an adverse effect on sensitive people.

Geopathic stress: Negative health effects on the body caused by geoelectromagnetic frequencies and earth energy disturbances. Geopathic stress may be caused by underground water, mining or construction activities, natural or manmade electromagnetic currents, or "dragon" (ley) lines crossing in the vicinity.

Grounded: Being grounded means you are fully present in incarnation, centered around your core, and solidly anchored in the current moment. It gives a feeling of relaxed certainty and being in control of yourself. You are aware and in touch with the planet, able to function within the practical, everyday world and yet able to extend into spiritual awareness as appropriate.

Positive DNA potential: Presently, 97 percent of DNA is identified as "non-functioning," but studies of so-called "junk DNA" show that it contains memories of personal trauma and transgenerational memories, which affect both the karmic blueprint and our subtle energy fields. This has enormous implications for our health, well-being, and evolution. But the good news is that the potential exists to switch off this outdated detrimental genetic coding (including ancestral inheritance) and to switch on beneficial codes to bring about changes in physical, mental, and emotional functioning—like upgrading the random access memory in a computer, having first deconstructed and removed outdated programs and remnants of former programs.

Sick-building syndrome: A condition caused by a building with air pollution, inadequate ventilation, excess static electricity, electromagnetic smog, geopathic stress, or related issues. Symptoms include lack of concentration, headache, chest and skin problems, nausea, excessive fatigue, and dizziness.

Ungrounded: Ungroundedness is the opposite of being grounded. When someone is ungrounded, he or she has only a toehold in incarnation, being unattached to the world and everyday reality. He or she is impractical, airheaded, forgetful, inattentive, and disconnected; he or she feels insecure, lacks a sense of control, and probably suffers from hyper-anxiety.

RESOURCES

PUBLICATIONS BY JUDY HALL

101 Power Crystals
The Crystal Bible (Volumes 1–3).
London: Godsfield Press Ltd, 2013.

The Crystal Companion

The Crystal Experience: Your Complete Crystal Workshop in a Book

Crystal Prescriptions (Volumes 1–6)

The Crystal Wisdom Healing Oracle

Crystals and Sacred Sites

Earth Blessings

The Encyclopedia of Crystals

Good Vibrations

Judy Hall's Book of Psychic Development

Life-Changing Crystals

Psychic Self-Protection

Crystals to Empower You

Crystal Love

CRYSTAL CLEANSING AND RECHARGING SPRAYS

Crystal Balance,
www.crystalbalance.co.uk

Green Man Shop,
www.greenmanshop.co.uk

Krystal Love,
www.krystallove.com.au

Petaltone Essences (United Kingdom),
www.petaltone.co.uk

Petaltone Essences
(United States of America),
www.petaltoneusa.com

Petaltone Essences (Japan),
www.petaltone-jp.com

Spiritual Planet,
www.spiritualplanet.co.uk

CRYSTALS

Exquisite Crystals
www.exquisitecrystals.com
John van Rees

Astrologywise
www.astrologywise.co.uk
Judy Hall

ACKNOWLEDGMENTS

I would like to thank Michael Illas for his skill, care, and sensitivity when photographing the crystals and layouts and all the workshop participants who have assisted in earth healing and grid work over the years and who have taught me so much. I much appreciated Yulia Surnina's assistance in setting out some of the grids and sorting through my crystal treasure trove. Many thanks go to Megan Buckley.

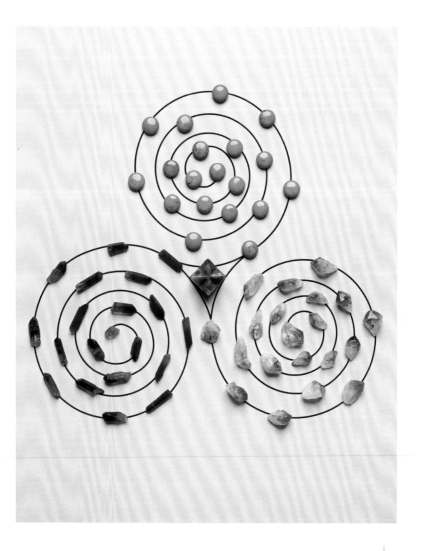

ABOUT THE AUTHOR

JUDY HALL (Dorset, England) is a successful Mind-Body-Spirit author with more than forty-seven MBS books to her credit including the million-copy selling *Crystal Bible* (volumes 1, 2, and 3), *101 Power Crystals, Crystals and Sacred Sites, Crystal Prescriptions,* and The *Crystal Wisdom Healing Oracle*. A trained healer and counselor, Judy has been psychic all her life and has a wide experience of many systems of divination and natural healing methods. Judy has a B.Ed in Religious Studies with an extensive knowledge of world religions and mythology and an M.A. in Cultural Astronomy and Astrology at Bath Spa University. Her expertise are past life readings and regression; soul healing, reincarnation, astrology and psychology, divination, and crystal lore. Judy has appeared four times in the Watkins list of the 100 most influential spiritual living writers and was voted the 2014 Kindred Spirit MBS personality of the year. An internationally known author, psychic, and healer, Judy conducts workshops in her native England and internationally. Her books have been translated into nineteen languages.

INDEX